NURSES' GUIDE TO TELEPHONE TRIAGE AND HEALTH CARE

NURSES' GUIDE TO TELEPHONE TRIAGE AND HEALTH CARE

GROUP HEALTH COOPERATIVE OF PUGET SOUND

A NURSECO BOOK

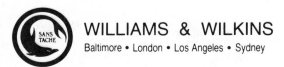

WILLIAMS & WILKINS
Baltimore • London • Los Angeles • Sydney

A NURSECO Book
Copyright © 1984
Margo Creighton Neal

Copyright © 1985
Williams & Wilkins
428 East Preston Street
Baltimore, MD 21202, U.S.A.

Printed in the United States of America

Library of Congress Cataloging in Publication Data

Main entry under title:

Nurses' guide to telephone triage and health care.

  Bibliography: p.
  1. Nursing. 2. Diagnosis. 3. Telephone—Emergency reporting systems. I. Group Health Cooperative of Puget Sound. [DNLM: 1. Emergency medical services—Nursing tests. 2. Emergency medical services—Handbooks. 3. Telephone—Handbooks. 4. Telephone—Nursing texts. WY 154 N9735]
RT48.N86   1983 616.02'4'024613   83-13373

ISBN 0-683-09526-9

85 86 87 88 89   10 9 8 7 6 5 4 3

CONTENTS

Adult Health Problems

CONTENTS

CONTENTS

Pediatric Health Problems

CONTENTS

FOREWORD

Over the past decade, the nurse has emerged as a provider of primary care. One of the expanded responsibilities of the primary care nurse is that of triage, which was initially a means of screening sick, wounded, or injured persons during wars or other disasters to help determine priority needs. This process helped to ensure effective use of medical and nursing manpower, equipment, and facilities.

Triaging is no longer limited to disaster and war, but has become a useful tool in everyday clinical practice. The focus of triage today is to help clients obtain appropriate care for their problems. The triage nurse interacts with clients and families, assesses presenting complaints, and intervenes with appropriate counseling and referrals.

Clients present with numerous complaints, and the triage nurse must accurately screen them in a short time period. Many nurses have been placed in this new role with little or no special preparation. Screening tools and resource materials must be readily available for them.

Nurses' Guide to Telephone Triage and Health Care is such a tool. It is designed to help nurses assess clients accurately and expediently. Protocols (guidelines) are provided for both adult and pediatric clients; common problems and complaints are indexed, and questions are identified to help the nurse establish an accurate history so that an initial assessment can be made. Clients then are referred for immediate attention or nonemergency follow-up; self-care and/or over-the-counter treatments can be recommended.

Quality triaging benefits both clients and health care providers. Clients are given guidance and direction in obtaining care from appropriate providers. This is especially welcomed by the consumer because of the high costs of medical care. In addition, health care providers can use their time and expertise more efficiently when clients have been properly screened. Protocols included in *Nurses' Guide to Telephone Triage and Health Care* are designed to help ensure consistent, accurate, quality triaging, thereby benefiting both clients and health care providers.

Linda La Plante, MSN, ANP
Associate Professor of Nursing
California State Univeristy, Los Angeles

Spiralling costs of health care today have stimulated development of a variety of approaches for delivering quality medical care efficiently and at a reduced cost. Telephone triage by registered nurses is one approach.

Nurses' Guide to Telephone Triage and Health Care was developed out of a need for concise telephone protocols (guidelines) designed to allow registered nurses and nurse practitioners to triage incoming telephone calls from clients. This component of health care delivery is time saving and cost-effective for both health care consumers and providers.

These telephone protocols, developed to augment the educational background of registered nurses, give specific, medically approved protocols for providing safe, effective telephone triage on a number of adult and pediatric health problems. The problems have been selected for one or more of the following reasons:

—they occur frequently in outpatient care and often are amenable to home treatment without physician intervention

—they are urgent or emergent health care problems that require skilled nursing assessment and intervention to assure a better outcome for the client

—they are health care problems for which a diagnosis has been established already by a physician, but about which the client is seeking more information

—they are problems that require referral for medical intervention.

The *Nurses' Guide to Telephone Triage and Health Care* is easy to use and provides:

- a standard of triage
- consistent advice and guidelines
- a combination of medical and nursing information
- specific home treatments
- information on pediatric dosages of commonly used medications
- color-coded, alphabetical entries and extensive cross-references
- a glossary of terms.

A substantial amount of time is spent by registered nurses responding to consumers' telephone requests for health advice and information. The role of the registered nurse pertaining to telephone health care is clear. The nurse *gathers needed information in the most accurate manner possible to guarantee a safe disposition of the problem*. This goal can be achieved by the following nursing process:

1. The nurse *assesses* the problem by listening to the caller's explanation and by eliciting information in a systematic manner.
2. The nurse makes *nursing diagnosis* by synthesizing the client's signs and symptoms, the client's reaction to the problem (e.g., anxiety, avoidance, hesitancy), the nurse's own knowledge, the information from the individual protocols, and the urgency and severity of the problem.
3. The nurse prescribes *intervention*, which may include health teaching, advice for a specific treatment approach, reassurance, or direction to a medical facility.
4. *Evaluation* of the nursing action is primarily up to the client. The client can call back if home treatment is unsuccessful or the situation worsens; in some instances, the nurse may instruct the caller to call back in a specified period of time. Thus, each step of the nursing process is utilized in telephone triage.

Nurses' Guide to Telephone Triage and Health Care is not a diagnostic tool, nor does it provide complete protocols for the management of each client problem. Rather, it alerts the registered nurse to ramifications of the problem, assists the nurse in making an accurate assessment, and provides guidelines for effective treatment alternatives.

PREFACE

The information contained in *Nurses' Guide to Telephone Triage and Health Care* has been derived from the working knowledge of nurses experienced in providing telephone health care, nurse clinical specialists, physicians, and reference texts. The protocols can be adapted to suit any facility that provides such a service.

The *Nurses' Guide to Telephone Triage and Health Care* was developed by Group Health Cooperative for use by registered nurses within the Group Health Cooperative System. Group Health Cooperative of Puget Sound is not responsible for the use of the protocols by any individual other than a Group Health Cooperative registered nurse. Any person, institution, or organization using these guidelines assumes full responsibility for acts or omissions arising out of their use.

Consultation with medical staff when a problem arises that is beyond the scope of nursing is mandated by law. Further legal implications may be imposed by the Nurse Practice Act of the state in which the nurse is practicing. Individuals using this book need to be aware of the legal guidelines that define the area of practice and the extent to which they regulate the use of this work.

Finally, we have attempted to avoid stereotyping the nurse as "she" and the client as "he" by using "s/he" whenever possible. However, the English language has yet to produce a combination form for masculine and feminine pronouns, thus you will note some referral to the client in the masculine or feminine form only.

Group Health Cooperative of Puget Sound

ACKNOWLEDGMENTS

Many people contributed directly and indirectly to this resource manual. We wish to recognize the nursing and medical staffs of Group Health Cooperative, particularly the consulting nurses in the Central Hospital Emergency Department, for the material contained in this book. The consulting nurses worked diligently in collaboration with other consulting nurses in the Cooperative to complete the project.

We also acknowledge Mary Gruenewald, RN, BSN, project director and originator of the concept of the consulting nurse role, for her long-term commitment to the project, and Karen Artz, RN, MS, editor and contributor to the work. We appreciate the clinical experience she brought to the project.

Other contributors we wish to acknowledge include Vernon Ross, MD, consulting editor, Robert Hauck, MD, Darrell Halverson, MD, Constance Macdonald, MD, and Gayle Thout, MD, for their critique and contributions; Linda Felthous, RPh, for reviewing the medication dosages, the Consulting Nurse Task Force, and Jeanine Schneider and Clara Moon for their assistance and expertise in preparing the original manuscript.

This book is dedicated to all these professionals in grateful recognition of their special contributions.

Group Health Cooperative of Puget Sound

The *Nurses' Guide to Telephone Triage and Health Care* is divided into two sections: adult health problems and pediatric health problems. The problems are arranged in alphabetical order within each section; extensive cross-references are included. The format for each problem has several distinct components:

Definition Describes the problem.

Etiology Refers to the common causes of the problem. It is not an all-inclusive list.

Assessment Information included in this section is variable. For some entries, symptoms are listed. It may also include factors that differentiate one problem from another, if both show similar symptoms. Information may be provided to assist in ruling out possible alternative diagnoses.

Teaching/ Treatment Defines treatment items that can be used in the home to 1) resolve the problem, 2) offer palliative treatment, 3) provide guidelines to teach the client about the condition, or 4) provide temporary or emergency care until medical help is available.

Refer to MD Defines when the client needs to be seen in a physician's office or a walk-in emergency department (if there is a need to evaluate a condition after clinic hours, but there is no life-threatening situation).

Emergency Defines either when a situation should be considered an emergency or what action to take in an emergency.

Cross Reference Lists other problems or treatments that pertain to client's problem.

In addition to the information provided, every card is *color coded* to alert the nurse to particular aspects of care needing special emphasis:
Yellow—signifies information that should be given to the client or caller
Orange—indicates the need for physician evaluation
Red—signals the need for emergency care.
Telephone assessment is a difficult task for many reasons. One of the most frustrating reasons is that the nurse cannot see or touch the client but must rely on information that either the client or an observer provides and on the nurse's "gut feeling" and auditory sense. The telephone nurse consultant rarely speaks with an observer who has a medical background and skills or access to the client's record or chart. Therefore, the nurse must gather information in the most accurate manner possible to guarantee safe disposition of the problem.
To use the *Nurses' Guide to Telephone Triage and Health Care* most effectively, we suggest that you first scan the Table of Contents to discover the adult and pediatric problems that are included; second, study the format of the protocols, noting the composition of each component; and lastly, study the following guidelines, which are based on the cumulative experience of the telephone triage nurses at Group Health Cooperative:
1. Greet the client in a calm manner, identify your role and willingness to help. For example, "This is the Consulting Nurse. May I help you?"
2. If several calls come in at the same time, do not put a client on hold until you have established that it is not an emergency and the client can, in fact, hold for a few minutes.

3. Talk directly to the client whenever possible. Observers or family may interpret the situation much differently than the client. Even children age eight and above can describe their problems quite accurately.
4. Let the client be the "expert" during the initial phase of the conversation. At this time, you will have no idea what the problem is and will get the best information by listening. Then, as the problem is explored and defined and disposition is determined, you will become the "expert."
5. Elicit information rather than solicit responses. Ask open-ended questions, for example, "Tell me what your pain feels like." This will produce more valuable information than, "Is it a crushing pain?" If the client is unable to describe the problem, offer some alternatives such as: "Is it like a knife stabbing you? Is it like pins and needles? Is it steady or does it come and go?" Try to get the client to describe the problem in his or her own words. Sometimes reminding clients that you cannot see them and must rely on their information will produce more descriptive data.
6. Respond to the client's anxiety. Even though the presenting symptoms may seem minor to you, if the caller is very anxious and you are not able to decrease the anxiety, suggest that the client be seen at a medical facility.
7. You have a limited number of senses with which to gather data; learn to trust your "gut reaction." If you feel uneasy about a client, have the client come in for evaluation.
8. If the client has a language barrier or accent that makes it difficult for you to communicate and evaluate the problem, advise the client to come in.
9. Telephone assessment of infants is very difficult. Tell the caller to bring the infant, especially those under six months, to the medical facility for evaluation.
10. Ensure that the caller understands any instructions given for treatment by asking the caller to repeat the information. "Do you understand?" is not an accurate way to assess if the caller understands the directions.
11. Determine if the caller is satisfied that the nurse has assessed the problem accurately and has given appropriate advice, e.g., "Do you feel comfortable with my assessment of the problem and can you follow the advice that I've given?" If the caller is not satisfied, offer the option for the client to come in.
12. Always allow the client to be evaluated in person in lieu of or instead of home treatment.
13. Tell the client to call back if the situation worsens or establish some time limit within which the client is to call if home treatment is unsuccessful. For example, "Call back in 30 minutes if using the hot water bottle has not relieved your pain or call sooner if the pain gets worse."
14. **The registered nurse is primarily responsible for assessing the urgency and severity of the problem and for providing an appropriate disposition based on that assessment**. Consult with the medical staff when a problem arises that is beyond your skill, training, and responsibility.
15. Document the telephone encounter identifying the client's name, age, and phone number (especially important, since the nurse may need to reestablish contact), chief complaint, major signs and symptoms, the *nursing assessment*, and the treatment alternatives provided. A sample form is provided in the appendix.

A sample documentation form is provided in Appendix 2, page 433.

In summary, telephone health care by the registered nurse is an acceptable form of health care delivery. The role of the nurse is to obtain information about the problem and provide safe and appropriate disposition. Legally, the role of the nurse is within the scope of nursing practice, particularly when compared to a community standard. The Telephone Guides can provide the community standard.

We welcome any comments or suggestions that you have regarding content, additions, or format. We hope that you find this *Nurses' Guide to Telephone Triage and Health Care* a dynamic, vital addition to your nursing practice.

ADULT
HEALTH
PROBLEMS

Discomfort in the abdominal area

Etiology See individual reference cards

Assessment Determine location, duration, intensity, onset, frequency, associated symptoms, history of similar problem, things that exacerbate or relieve it, character of pain, radiation of pain, presence or absence of fever, other contributing factors (e.g., possible onset of labor in pregnant woman, menstruation), client's medications.

Treatment/ Teaching May use heat (hot water bottle, heating pad, hot bath) for 20 to 30 minutes. Recontact nurse if no relief or discomfort increases.

Refer to MD If pain gradually increasing in intensity; of long duration; if fever present

Emergency If pain is constant, localized, unrelieved, rapidly increasing in intensity; client in severe distress

Cross Reference **With vomiting**: Appendicitis; Blood in Vomitus; Diabetic Ketoacidosis; Food Poisoning; Gall Bladder Colic; Gastroenteritis; Hepatitis; Kidney Stones; Obstruction, Intestinal; Salmonella Infection; Ulcer, Duodenal and Gastric; Urinary Tract Infection

Without vomiting: Abortion, Aneurysm, Belching, Bloating, Colitis, Constipation, Diarrhea, Dysmenorrhea, Ectopic Pregnancy, Gas, Giardiasis, Hiatus Hernia, Indigestion, Pelvic Inflammatory Disease, Stomach Ache

Expulsion from the uterus of the products of conception before viability (usually 24 weeks); may be spontaneous, threatened, or therapeutic

Etiology Intentional, ovular defects due to maternal or paternal factors, maternal trauma, infections, dietary deficiencies, diabetes mellitus, hypothroidism, poisoning, anatomic malformations, unknown

Assessment Usual symptoms include vaginal bleeding in a pregnant woman before period of viability, uterine cramping, disappearance of signs and symptoms of pregnancy; products of conception may or may not be expelled. R/o ruptured ectopic pregnancy, anovulatory bleeding in non-pregnant woman, membranous dysmenorrhea.

Treatment/ Teaching

Threatened abortion: Bedrest. Check if client has IUD. Be seen for heavy bleeding (saturating a pad every 2 hours or less), passage of tissue, or if fever or pain. Warm water bottle to abdomen for 30 minutes. If no relief, to be seen immediately.

Therapeutic abortion: Can be done up to 24 weeks gestation, usually before 20 weeks. May have diminishing flow for 2 weeks after procedure. Identify appropriate referral resources for the procedure.

Refer to MD For exam after spontaneous abortion, preparation for therapeutic abortion, evaluation of vaginal bleeding in early pregnancy

Emergency Heavy vaginal bleeding, passage of tissue, fever, pain, syncope

Cross Reference Abdominal Pain, Dysmenorrhea, Ectopic Pregnancy, Fever, Menorrhagia, Rho Gam Guidelines, Spotting

Superficial injury to skin or mucous membrane from scraping or rubbing

Etiology   Trauma to affected area

Assessment   Circumstances of injury, extent of wound, amount of bleeding

Treatment/ Teaching   Stop bleeding with pressure. Wash well with soap and water, remove all ingrained dirt, rinse off. Apply antibiotic ointment (e.g., Bacitracin) tid for 3 days. Apply dressing prn. Check for current tetanus immunization; if there has been none in past 5 years, immunize within 72 hours.

Refer to MD   If signs of infection appear in wound

Emergency   Large abrasion from barnyard area (high risk for tetanus)

Cross Reference   Bites, Animal and Human (Peds); Wound Infection

Condition occurring when a normally implanted placenta begins to separate from the uterus prior to delivery of the fetus

Etiology   Unknown

Assessment   Determine expected date of delivery. Usual symptoms include uterine pain, shock, vaginal bleeding (may or may not be present depending on the location of the separation) in late pregnancy.

Treatment/ Teaching   Refer to MD immediately

Refer to MD   To be seen immediately

Emergency   Uterine hemorrhage, shock

Cross Reference   Shock, Vaginal Hemorrhage

Skin condition in which blackheads are associated with papular and pustular eruption of pilosebaceous follicles

Etiology   Attributable to effect of androgenic hormones on pilosebaceous apparatus; affects 80% of teenagers, more common in males

Assessment   Distinguish from lesions caused by exposure to chemicals (e.g., bromides, iodides, contact with chlorinated napthalines and diphenyls).

Treatment/ Teaching

1. Gently, frequently degrease face with water and soap often enough to keep face dry and skin tight and oil free.

2. Apply acne lotion (per Rx from MD) at bedtime to all skin areas involved. If client does not have Rx from MD, may try a preparation containing benzyl peroxide (e.g., Benzyl Peroxide 4%, Acneeveen, Desquam-x Wash, Fostex Cream, Donax). NOTE: dryness and tightness are expected; if skin becomes red, sore, or chapped, stop applying lotion for 1 to 2 days and then resume.

3. Lather or shampoo hair daily; if dandruff shampoo used, let lather remain for 5 to 10 minutes before rinsing. May use conditioner on dry hair.

4. No special diet or diet restrictions; eat well-balanced diet.

5. Get adequate amount of rest (6 to 8 hours sleep/night).

6. Do not squeeze or pick lesions.

7. Do not expect much improvement for 2 to 3 months. Acne treatment is slow, but it works.

Refer to MD   For evaluation or if chapping persists with use of acne lotion

Emergency

Cross Reference   Pimples

Etiology

Assessment

**Treatment/
Teaching**

Refer to MD

Emergency

**Cross
Reference**

Anaphylaxis

An altered or exaggerated susceptibility to various foreign substances or physical agents that are harmless to the great majority of individuals.

Etiology Exposure to allergen (e.g., pollens, dust, medicines or serums, animals or insects, chemicals, foods)

Assessment Manifested in many ways including hay fever, asthma, hives, urticaria. Establish exposure to known allergen, history of allergies; determine extent of reaction (local vs systemic).

Treatment/ Teaching Oral antihistamines (e.g., diphenhydramine [Benadryl] or chlorpheniramine maleate [CTM]; check if client has on hand. Do not give antihistamines if client is hypertensive. Cold compresses, soda compresses, cool bath, Calamine lotion prn for urticaria. Discontinue suspected medication if drug related. Fluids prn for internal allergen (food or medicine).

Refer to MD If drug related or for evaluation and/or desensitization or hyposensitization to allergen

Emergency Anaphylactic reaction (i.e., generalized urticaria, parasthesia, choking, cyanosis, wheezing, shock, loss of consciousness, convulsions, fever, cough, incontinence, facial edema)

Cross Reference Allergy Shot Reaction, Anaphylaxis, Asthma, Hay fever, Hives, Sinus Congestion

Local or systemic response following the administration of desensitizing or hyposensitizing vaccines

Etiology Injection of known antigen

Assessment History of allergies with recent (within past several hours) immunization for allergies

Treatment/ Teaching Oral antihistamines (e.g., diphenhydramine [Benadryl] or chlorpheniramine [CTM]). Ice pack locally to reduce swelling. Decrease activity and exposure to allergens. Client to remain in MD's office for 20 minutes after injection. Measure size of red area (flare) to report to MD. Note: Oral antihistamines **should not** be taken before immunization.

Refer to MD To report reaction

Emergency Anaphylactic reaction (will occur within 20 minutes; first signs are sneezing, coughing, chest tightness and/or generalized flush, tingling sensations, pruritis)

Cross Reference Allergies, Anaphylaxis, Ice Pack (Glossary), Wheezing

Cessation of menses (temporarily or permanently)

Etiology   Pregnancy, "silent period," illness, travel, menopause, emotional stress, malnutrition, anemia, lactation, cessation of birth control pills, pituitary tumors

Assessment   Rely on history and ancillary symptoms. R/o pregnancy, menopause.

Treatment/ Teaching   If client is on birth control pills and has taken all her pills, but has no period at the end of the cycle, this may be a "silent period." Continue to take the pills as usual, contact MD if no period occurs after the second cycle. If pregnancy suspected, can do a pregnancy urine or blood test 6 weeks (42 days) after the first day of the last menstrual period. If amemorrhea occurs without the use of birth control pills, client should contact MD if regular period not reestablished in next cycle.

Refer to MD   For repeated, missed periods, for evaluation of underlying problem

Emergency

Cross Reference   Anemia; Birth Control Pills; Menopausal Syndrome; Menstrual Problems; Pregnancy, Diagnosis of

An acute, often explosive reaction occurring in a previously sensitized person

Etiology Foreign serum, certain drugs or diagnostic agents, desensitizing injections, insect stings

Assessment Typically, in 1 to 15 minutes after exposure to the allergen, the client complains of a sense of uneasiness, becomes agitated, flushed. Palpitations, paresthesias, pruritis, throbbing in the ears, coughing, sneezing, difficulty in breathing are other typical complaints. Signs and symptoms of shock may develop within another 1 or 2 minutes; the client may become incontinent, convulse, become unresponsive, and die. It is important to recognize early signs before shock develops; this client is flushed and has a rapid pulse, in contrast to the client with the more common vasovagal syncope who develops pallor and bradycardia.

Treatment/ Teaching Oral antihistamine, (e.g., diphenhydramine [Benadryl] or chlorpheniramine [CTM]) if readily available and if the client can swallow. Arrange emergency transportation to hospital.

Refer to MD Arrange emergency transportation to the hospital

Emergency Emergency aid STAT

Cross Reference Allergies, Bee Sting, Coma, Convulsions, Swallowing Difficulty, Wheezing

Disorder due to a deficiency in the number of red blood cells and/or their hemoglobin content

Etiology   Usually due to excessive blood loss (e.g., heavy menstrual flow, gastrointestinal bleeding), prolonged poor diet.

Assessment   Usual symptoms include pallor, lassitude, easy fatigability, irritability, dyspnea, palpitations, angina, tachycardia; often anorexia, compulsive eating of anything. Iron-deficiency anemia must be differentiated from other types of anemia. Determine cause, if possible (e.g., history of heavy periods, rectal bleeding, hematemesis, history of ulcers, hiatus hernia, excessive salicylate intake, bleeding hemorrhoids).

Treatment/ Teaching   Take prescribed iron preparations after meals to help avoid gastrointestinal upset. High-protein diet to increase iron intake through food (fish, meat [especially liver], iron-enriched bread and cereals, egg yolk, green vegetables, dried fruits).

Refer to MD   For evaluation and treatment

Emergency

Cross Reference   Amenorrhea, Angina, Fatigue, Palpitations

Rupture of a localized dilation of the aorta

Etiology

Defect in the arterial wall due to disease or injury

Assessment

R/o myocardial infarction. This type of chest pain does not usually radiate down the arms. Clients with ischemic heart disease usually lie quietly even though they report the pain to be intense. Clients suffering with acute aortic dissection are often restless and agitated. Pain is **sudden, severe, tearing**, frequently radiating to back between scapula; may progress to neck, chin, and even abdomen.

Treatment/ Teaching

Arrange emergency transportation to hospital.

Refer to MD

Emergency

Emergency transportation to hospital

Cross Reference

Abdominal Pain, Chest Pain, Pain in Side

Localized myocardial ischemia

Etiology   Often due to arteriosclerotic heart disease

Assessment   Sensation of pain, squeezing, burning, pressing, choking, aching, "gas," or tightness in chest appearing during exertion and increasing in intensity until the client rests. Pain is not sharp and localized, is of short duration, usually subsides completely without residual discomfort. Pain is retrosternal or slightly to the left and may radiate to one or both shoulders, arms, neck, and occasionally intrascapular area. It is especially aggravated by **cold weather activity**, exertion, eating, emotional stress.

**Treatment/
Teaching**   Instruct client to take nitroglycerine (NTG) as follows:

Take one. If no relief in 5 minutes, take another. If no relief in 5 minutes after the second one, take a third one. If no relief after 3, client needs emergency transportation to hospital.

Vasodilator drugs such as NTG should produce prompt relief; excessive dosage can cause headache or syncope. Tell client to take NTG while sitting (to help prevent syncope), and that s/he may also experience headache, facial flushing. NTG stings when placed under the tongue. A sudden, marked increase in the number of NTG required in a day may signal significant changes in cardiac status (e.g., unstable angina). NTG remains potent for 1 year in original container.

Refer to MD   For evaluation of first attack or attacks of increasing frequency, intensity, or duration

Emergency   If no relief after 3 nitroglycerin taken 5 minutes apart, arrange emergency transportation to hospital.

**Cross
Reference**   Anemia, Chest Pain, Palpitations

Lack of desire to eat

Etiology Infections, gastrointestinal disturbances, chronic illness, anorexia nervosa or other psychiatric problems, medications, endocrine disorder, central nervous system disease, anxiety, cancer, hepatitis

Assessment Most causes are transient and are not associated with significant metabolic changes. R/o prolonged problem resulting in significant weight loss or other serious ancillary symptoms.

Treatment/ Teaching Clear fluids and foods as tolerated. Watch for any significant weight loss and/or signs of dehydration.

Refer to MD If problem persists longer than a few days

Emergency

Cross Reference Chemotherapy, Dehydration, Nausea and Vomiting

Guidelines for administration

Etiology

Assessment

There is an association, but not yet a proved causal relationship, between the use of aspirin in viral illnesses and subsequent Reye's Syndrome. Until this relationship is definitively established by the FDA, DO NOT recommend aspirin as the antipyretic agent of choice in viral illnesses, especially influenza and chickenpox (use acetaminophen instead).

Aspirin (ASA) is indicated for treatment of fever, pain, and inflammation. A common side effect is gastric distress. Acetaminophen is indicated for treatment of pain or fever; **it has no anti-inflammatory effect**. There are no significant side effects when given in therapeutic doses. Liver damage can result from overdosage.

Treatment/ Teaching

For teenagers through adulthood

Medication	How Supplied	Dosage
Aspirin (Bufferin, Anacin, Excedrin; all contain ASA as the active ingredient)	Usually 5 grs (300 mgm) per tablet. Some superstrength preparations are available; have caller read you the label for tablet strength.	10 grains (2 tablets) every 4 hours prn
Acetaminophen (Tylenol, Datril, Anacin 3)	Tablets: Usually 325 mgm; Capsules: Check strength with caller. Some superstrength preparations are available. Have caller read the label for pill strength.	10 grains (2 tablets) every 4 hours prn

Refer to MD

Emergency

Cross Reference

Aspirin and Acetaminophen (Peds)

A feeling of apprehension, uncertainty, or tension related to the individual's anticipation of a real or imagined threat to his mental or physical well-being

Etiology

Unknown, internal, related to the future, vague, or caused by psychologic conflict

Assessment

Symptoms include irritability, tenseness, impaired concentration, fearfulness, rapid pulse and respiration, sweating, insomnia, GI upset, dilated pupils, headache, palpitations, chest pain, restlessness, fatigue, dry mouth, and hyperventilation. When anxiety reaches a certain intensity, it becomes overwhelming and limits one's actions. Check if client is using any kind of drugs.

Treatment/ Teaching

Accept person's anxiety and do not judge; be supportive. Help client express concerns. Try to channel and direct energy of anxiety into activities (e.g., exercise, involvement with supportive friends, hot baths, deep-breathing exercises, jogging). Help client understand reasons for anxiety and explore possible solutions and ways to limit external stresses.

Refer to MD

If anxiety is overwhelming (state of panic); for evaluation of associated physical symptoms. Client may also be referred to a community mental health service for counseling.

Emergency

Cross Reference

Chest Pain, Hyperventilation, Insomnia, Shakiness

Inability to receive and/or send verbal messages

Etiology   CVA, brain tumor, cerebral aneurysm

Assessment   Rely on history and ancillary symptoms. Check for weakness, numbness, mobility, duration and type of aphasia, headache, recent injury, cyanosis or respiratory distress, level of consciousness.

Treatment/ Teaching   For previously diagnosed problem, instruct family members as follows:

1. Speak slowly and give short simple directions. Repeat if necessary.
2. Give client plenty of time to respond.
3. Face the client when talking so s/he can see your expressions. Gestures are helpful.
4. Be prepared for swearing or unusual language. Try not to react negatively if it occurs.
5. Emphasize the client's abilities.
6. Allow client to be as independent as possible. Find activities to create a feeling of usefulness.
7. Alert friends to problem before they visit to avoid embarrassing both them and the client.
8. Don't push client into attempts to read and write too soon.
9. Praise client for attempts to speak and for small gains.
10. Develop a communication system (e.g., flash cards, paper and pencil).

Refer to MD   For evaluation of a new problem, for evaluation and initiation of speech therapy of a previously diagnosed problem

Emergency   Sudden onset accompanied by respiratory distress, loss of muscle function

Cross Reference   Stroke

APPENDICITIS

Inflammation of the appendix

Etiology Obstruction of the appendiceal lumen by a fecalith, inflammation, foreign body, or neoplasm

Assessment Symptoms usually begin with epigastric or periumbilical pain associated with 1 to 2 episodes of vomiting. Within 2 to 12 hours, the pain shifts to the right lower quadrant and persists as a steady soreness that is aggravated by coughing or walking. Anorexia, moderate malaise, and slight fever are present. Constipation is usual, but diarrhea occurs occasionally. Acute gastroenteritis is most commonly confused with appendicitis. Mesenteric adenitis, Meckel's diverticulitis, regional enteritis, amebiasis, perforated duodenal ulcer, ureteral colic, acute salpingitis, mittelschmerz, ruptured ectopic pregnancy, and twisted ovarian cyst can also be confused with appendicitis. Ask if stepping down (i.e., off a stair or low stool) gives a jarring pain.

Treatment/ Teaching Nothing PO while evaluating condition. Try mild heat to abdomen for 30 to 45 minutes at home. Be seen if no relief.

Refer to MD If pain gradually increasing in intensity and unrelieved with heat

Emergency If pain is constant, localized, severe

Cross Reference Abdominal Pain, Fever, Nausea and Vomiting

Etiology

Assessment

Treatment/
Teaching

Refer to MD

Emergency

Cross
Reference   Atrial Fibrillation, Dysrhythmias, Paroxysmal Atrial Tachycardia

Degenerative joint disease

Etiology Predisposing factors include aging, obesity, and joint trauma

Assessment This is a degenerative disorder without systemic manifestations. It involves pain in 1 or more joints, is not crippling unless the hip is involved. More women are affected than men and onset usually occurs near menopause. Onset is insidious with articular stiffness initially and then pain with motion of the affected joint, which is made worse with prolonged activity and relieved by rest. Limitation of movement of the affected joints is common. Rheumatoid arthritis can be quite crippling, flares periodically, and is a different entity from osteoarthritis.

Treatment/ Teaching Rest the affected joint or joints, local heat (if hands affected, wrap in warm, moist towels for 20 minutes). Physical therapy and exercise as prescribed. ASA analgesics. If the client has had a cortisone injection, pain may be more severe within the first 24 hours. Use heat to the injection site to speed up absorption of drug and for comfort. Client may need codeine or other narcotic to manage pain initially.

Refer to MD For evaluation and for management of pain and inflammation

Emergency

Cross Reference Bursitis

Etiology

Assessment

**Treatment/
Teaching**

Refer to MD

Emergency

**Cross
Reference**   Choking, Pneumonia

ASPIRIN OVERDOSE

Ingestion of aspirin in excess of therapeutic dose

Etiology Intentional, accidental

Assessment History of ingestion of ASA accompanied by rapid, deep breathing, flushed face, hyperthermia, tinnitus, abdominal pain, vomiting, headache, profuse perspiration, restlessness, excitement, convulsions, or coma

Toxic Doses: Adults—0.4 to 0.5 Gm/kg (3 to 4 gr/lb). Quick Calculation: 1 tab (5 gr)/lb. CHILDREN ARE MORE SENSITIVE (leading cause of pediatric deaths by poisoning.) Baby Aspirin: 1 tab = 1/gr. Toxic dose for children same as for adults.

Treatment/ Teaching If ingestion occurred within past 6 hours, induce vomiting (using Ipecac per instructions according to body weight). Give 6 to 8 ounces of clear fluid (no red juice) before giving Ipecac. Call client back in 20 to 25 minutes to check that vomiting occurred. Nothing PO for 40 minutes after Ipecac, then diet as tolerated.

Refer to MD If no vomiting of aspirin occurred, if amount of ingestion is undetermined

Emergency If toxic symptoms present

Cross Reference Ipecac Protocol (Peds), Overdose, Poisoning

Obstruction of the flow of air in the smaller bronchi and bronchioles, manifested by recurrent paroxysms of dyspnea or characteristic wheezing

Etiology   Inherited allergic constitution, infection in the upper or lower respiratory tract, irritating inhalants, cold air, exercise, emotional upset

Assessment   Usual symptoms include recurrent attacks of dyspnea; cough; expectoration of tenacious, mucoid sputum; wheezing. Symptoms may be mild and occur only in association with respiratory infection, or may occur in varying degrees of severity to the point of being life threatening. Classical allergic asthma usually begins in childhood; can become progressively more severe throughout life. Spontaneous remissions may occur in adulthood. The acute attack is characterized by dyspnea, usually associated with an expiratory wheeze that may be heard without a stethoscope.

Treatment/ Teaching   Clear fluids. Vaporizer, steamy bathroom or out in night air (if cool and damp). Bronchodilator meds if previously prescribed for client (Tedral, Marax, Aminophylline can be taken every 4 hours around the clock prn to relieve wheezing; usual dose is QID; can increase dose to 6 times a day if needed to manage symptoms over a short period [i.e., 24 hours]). No decongestants with asthma medications (too drying to secretions).

Refer to MD   If unrelieved with home treatment; for evaluation of associated respiratory infection

Emergency   If severe respiratory distress present, especially any cyanosis

Cross Reference   Allergies, Cough, Cyanosis, Breathing Difficulty, Upper Respiratory Infection, Wheezing

ATELECTASIS

A shrunken and airless state of the lung, or part thereof, which may be acute or chronic, complete or incomplete

Etiology Bronchial obstruction causing resorption of alveolar air; postoperative immobility; presence of a foreign body, neoplasm, or mucus plug

Assessment **Acute:** Pain on affected side, sudden dyspnea and cyanosis, tachycardia, fever, shock, decreased chest motion.
Chronic: May be no signs other than x-ray abnormalities.

Treatment/ Teaching Often an emergency situation; may have a partial collapse of lung with dyspnea and moderate (not severe) pain; still needs to come to ER. Position of comfort until aid arrives; reassure client.

Refer to MD

Emergency For acute pain, dyspnea, shock; arrange emergency transportation to hospital

Cross Reference Chest Pain, Cyanosis, Fever

Pruritic, scaling lesions of feet due to fungus

Etiology Fungal invasion of the skin between the toes

Assessment Itching, burning, stinging of webs, palms, and soles. Deep vesicles in acute stage; fissuring, maceration in chronic stage. Distinguish from yeast infection, psoriasis, contact dermatitis, eczema, scabies. Rarely occurs before puberty.

Treatment/ Teaching Keep feet clean and dry. Apply antifungal medication (e.g., Desinex powder and ointment, Whitfield's ointment) daily. Wear cotton socks and change daily. Wear sandals or open-toed shoes; no tennis shoes. Wear rubber or wooden sandals in community showers or bathing places.

Refer to MD If no improvement with home treatment or if secondary infection develops

Emergency

Cross Reference Dermatitis, Fungal Infections

An irregular heart rhythm with a variable ventricular rate

Etiology
Rheumatic heart disease, especially mitral stenosis, and arteriosclerotic heart disease; infection, trauma, surgery, poisoning, or excessive alcohol intake may cause attacks in clients with normal hearts.

Assessment
Most common chronic dysrhythmia. It is the only common dysrhythmia in which the ventricular rate is rapid and the rhythm irregular. Check medications. Check for history of chronic heart problems. Some people have "slow" atrial fibrillation with a ventricular response in the normal range (i.e., 80 to 100). They need not be seen unless there is something new occurring and/or they are symptomatic. Most initial episodes of atrial fibrillation will be accompanied by chest tightness, breathlessness (not SOB or dyspneic), and palpitation resulting from anxiety caused by a new and different sensation to the client.

Treatment/ Teaching
Lie down; relax; breathe less than 12 times/minute.

Refer to MD

Emergency
Palpitations or dysrhythmia lasting longer than 10 minutes

Cross Reference
Dysrhythmias, Paroxysmal Atrial Tachycardia

Discomfort in the thoracic, sacral, lumbar, or coccygeal area of back

Etiology   Injury, structural inadequacy, intervertebral disk abnormality, specific disease of vertebrae, physiologic or abnormal function elsewhere in body, discomfort of pregnancy, onset of labor, UTI, positioning

Assessment   Rely on history and ancillary symptoms. Check for onset, intensity, frequency, and duration of the pain, history of trauma to area, presence of peripheral numbness, if pain radiates down leg below knee, what measures if any relieve the discomfort, presence of any loss of function of extremities, any relationship to pregnancy, presence of urinary tract symptoms. Suspect herniated disk if client stands tilted to one side or is unable to resume total upright posture.

Treatment/ Teaching   **Muscle strain or spasm**: Bedrest, maximum 1 to 2 days. Should become easier to move with less pain. Lie on side in fetal position to relax muscles or on back with small pillow under head and 1 to 2 pillows under knees. Ice for 20 to 30 minutes every 2 hours for 48 hours. ASA prn.

UTI or pregnancy: See cross reference cards.

Refer to MD   If no relief with home treatment or for evaluation of cause if problem is chronic

Emergency   Severe pain, possible spinal fracture, spinal cord injury

Cross Reference   Ice Massage (Glossary); Muscle Pain or Spasm; Pregnancy, Minor Discomforts of; Strain; UTI

Offensive breath odor

Etiology Improper oral hygiene, chronic nasal and sinus disease, dental caries, gum infections, tonsillar infections, chronic pulmonary disease or abscess, gastrointestinal disease, offensive foods (e.g., onions, garlic), dentures

Assessment

Treatment/ Teaching Good dental care, oral hygiene. Antiseptic mouthwashes or saline gargles. Decongestants for postnasal drip (e.g., pseudoephedrine [Sudafed], chlortrimeton, [CTM]). Avoid offensive foods.

Refer to MD For evaluation and treatment if unrelieved by home treatment or due to infection

Emergency Any history suggesting pulmonary etiology (e.g., aspiration)

Cross Reference Saline Gargle (Glossary)

Difficulty in maintaining upright posture; may be associated with dizziness

Etiology CVA, alcohol intoxication, medications, inner ear infection, head injury, muscle weakness, chronic disease, high fever, orthostatic hypotension, hypoglycemia, hyperventilation, seizure disorder

Assessment Rely on history and ancillary symptoms.

Treatment/ Teaching Appropriate to cause; see specific cross reference card.

Refer to MD For chronic and previously diagnosed problem, if sudden onset and/or severe intensity, if unrelieved with specific home treatment

Emergency If associated with onset of sudden paralysis or any other symptoms of stroke

Cross Reference Convulsions, Dizziness, Ear Infection, Fainting, Fever, Head Injury, Hyperventilation, Hypoglycemia, Stroke

Painful sensation caused by a bite or sting from a bee or other insect

Etiology

Assessment Known contact with bee or other insect. Area will look red and swollen and a little worse than a mosquito bite.

Treatment/ Teaching Remove stinger with flick of fingernail, do not squeeze. Apply baking soda or meat tenderizer paste (for 10 minutes, then rinse off) to help draw out stinger and poison sac. Use Calamine lotion, elevate area involved (swelling will be more predominant on the second day). Apply ice pack for 24 hours, then warm soaks. Initiate oral antihistamine (e.g., Benadryl, CTM) if client has known allergy to bee stings. Observe for allergic reaction. Watch for signs of infection, (i.e., redness, swelling, streaking)

Refer to MD If onset of systemic allergic symptoms is slow and mild or if secondary infection or cellulitis is present

Emergency Anaphylactic reaction

Cross Reference Anaphylaxis, Cellulitis, Meat Tenderizer Paste (Glossary), Wound Infection

Ejection of wind or gas spasmodically from the stomach through the mouth

Etiology   GI upset, hiatus hernia, diet containing gaseous foods

Assessment   Check for presence or absence of abdominal pain, problems with digestion, history of hiatus hernia, pregnancy.

Treatment/ Teaching   Eat small portions of food. Avoid highly spiced foods and gas-producing foods (e.g., beans, cabbage, cucumbers). Use antacids with simethicone (e.g., Digel, Mylanta II). Sit in an upright position. Put 3" to 4" blocks under head of bed if hiatus hernia present. Avoid eating within 2 hours of bedtime.

Refer to MD   For evaluation of chronic problem or if no relief with home treatment

Emergency

Cross Reference   Abdominal Pain, Gas, Hiatus Hernia, Indigestion

A form of mononeuritis involving the facial nerve

Etiology   Unknown in the majority of cases; sometimes precipitated by exposure, chill, or trauma

Assessment   Paralysis of muscles of 1 side of the face; pain is rarely present; often a feeling of stiffness of muscles on affected side

Treatment/ Teaching   Prompt treatment will usually shorten the recovery period. Reassure that recovery usually occurs in 2 to 8 weeks. Keep face warm, avoid exposure to wind and dust. Protect eye with patch if necessary; use artificial tears prn to keep cornea lubricated.

Refer to MD   For initial evaluation and follow-up

Emergency

Cross Reference   Numbness, Paralysis

Identification of the various ways to prevent conception

Etiology

Assessment

Types include birth control pills, IUD, diaphragm, foam, condoms, and rhythm

Treatment/ Teaching

Type	Advantages	Disadvantages
Birth Control Pills	99% effective; convenient. Produce regular, short, light periods. Low cost.	Minor side effects (nausea, breast tenderness, menstrual disturbances, headaches). Possible major side effects (e.g., thromboembolism, myocardial infarction, gall bladder disease, stroke) occur infrequently and are attributed to the pill only statistically. Incidence of major side effects increases over 35 years of age. Changes in metabolism of sugar. **Increased risk of embolism with smoking.**
IUD	Convenient, relatively high effectiveness (97%)	Side effects: heavier menses, prolonged menses in most women, dysmenorrhea; possibility of expulsion, increased incidence of PID, possibility of perforation requiring surgical removal. Higher incidence of ectopic pregnancy, midtrimester pregnancy sepsis, spontaneous abortion. Should be removed in early pregnancy. Higher incidence of problems during lactation.

Treatment/ Teaching continued	Diaphragm	About 97% effective. No side effects unless allergic to spermicide. Provides some protection against venereal disease.	Must be fit for size. Needs to be inserted prior to coitus and left in place at least 6 hours after intercourse. Additional jelly must be used if intercourse occurs more than 6 hours after placement of diaphragm and with each repeated intercourse. Some foams will disintegrate rubber. Check diaphragm for holes.
	Foam/Spermicidal Suppositories	Easy to insert. No side effects except occasional allergy (of the woman or her partner). Some protection against venereal disease.	Needs to be inserted prior to each act of coitus. Higher failure rate (about 95% effective).
	Condoms	Effectiveness 95%. Excellent protection against venereal disease. No side effects.	Must be put on before coitus. Occasional failures. Rare allergy to rubber.
	Foam and Condoms	Excellent effectiveness (99%). Excellent protection against venereal disease.	Put on/insert before coitus. Rare allergy to foam. Some foams will disintegrate rubber.
	Rhythm	No side effects. No special precautions required at time of coitus.	Impractical for women with irregular menses. High failure rate. Effectiveness around 85% for women with fairly regular cycles using conventional rhythm method. Effectiveness high for women with regular cycles using Billings' and ovulation methods. Requires large amount of instruction and practice, intelligent user, high motivation to abstain at appropriate times during the cycle.

Refer to MD   For information and/or insertion of birth control device

Emergency

Cross Reference   Birth Control Pills, Vasectomy

Directions for use and problems that are commonly encountered with use

Etiology

Assessment

Treatment/
Teaching
In initiating course, use foam and/or condoms during first month, especially if pills started after 7th day of cycle. If caller
- missed 1 pill, reassure; take pill as soon as she remembers, then continue as usual unless several days have gone by.
- missed 1 pill several days ago, continue as usual.
- missed 2 pills, take pills bid for 2 days then continue full number of days (use new package).
- took dose at a different time, continue as usual
- missed 3 or more days, begin using other form of contraception, stop pills and restart in 1 week for full cycle.
- missed pills at beginning of cycle, restart cycle as usual (will throw cycle off by same number of days missed); use other form of contraception for 2 weeks.

Client is infertile from 1st day as long as entire cycle is completed (except for 1st month on the pill). When stopping pill, use another form of contraception and wait 2 months before trying to conceive.

Refer to MD
If nausea, vomiting, fluid retention, or other side effects result from taking the pill

Emergency

Cross
Reference
Amenorrhea, Birth Control Methods, Break-Through Bleeding

Etiology Animal and human

Assessment

**Treatment/
Teaching**

Refer to MD

Emergency

**Cross
Reference** Bites, Animal and Human (Peds); Rabies

Black coloration in feces

Etiology Gastrointestinal bleeding, ingestion of certain foods and drugs

Assessment Check for presence of abdominal pain, history of ulcers, or other source of GI bleeding, alcoholism, presence of hematemesis, recent ingestion of beets, iron pills, Pepto Bismol. Check if client is on Coumadin, steroids, aspirin, Indocin, phenylbutazone.

Treatment/ Teaching Suspect GI bleeding. If client asymptomatic after 1 stool, instruct to contact MD. If symptom related to food, iron therapy, or Pepto Bismol, reassure.

Refer to MD For evaluation of problem if client asymptomatic or experiencing mild discomfort

Emergency If symptom accompanied by severe abdominal pain, hematemesis, rectal bleeding, dizziness, or lightheadedness

Cross Reference Abdominal Pain; Blood in Vomitus; Blood in Stools; Rectal Bleeding; Ulcer, Duodenal and Gastric

Black discoloration to tongue

Etiology Some food combinations (e.g., licorice, blueberries), side effect of some antibiotics, liquid iron, Pepto Bismol

Assessment Rely on diet and medication history, ancillary symptoms.

Treatment/ Teaching Discontinue antibiotic temporarily (if seems to be the cause) and contact MD. Increase fluids.

Refer to MD For evaluation and treatment if cause is unknown or if medication change is necessary

Emergency

Cross Reference

Discomfort or pain in the area of the bladder

Etiology   Acute urinary retention or distention of a bladder wall altered by tuberculosis or interstitial cystitis; bladder infection

Assessment   Pain caused by **overdistention** is relieved by emptying the bladder. Pain due to **bladder infection** is usually referred to the distal urethra and accompanies micturition. Check for presence of hematuria, burning, frequency, urgency, fever, decreased urinary output.

Treatment/ Teaching   Attempt to void. This may be made easier by voiding in a warm tub bath (warmth will help relax the bladder muscle). Increase fluids.

Refer to MD   If unable to void in an 8 to 12 hour period; for extreme pain, fever, abdominal distention

Emergency

Cross Reference   Blood in Urine; Burning on Urination; Voiding Difficulty; Fever; Urine, Decreased Output or Stream

Etiology

Assessment

Treatment/
Teaching

Refer to MD

Emergency

Cross
Reference   Bladder Pain; Bed Wetting (Peds); Blood in Urine; Burning on Urination; Voiding Difficulty;
Incontinence, Urinary; Nocturia; Urine, Decreased Output or Stream

Guidelines for evaluating hematuria after dilatation procedure

Etiology   Trauma from procedure

Assessment   History of recent procedure

Treatment/ Teaching   Expect some bleeding for 24 hours after procedure. Bedrest. Fluids. If stream is clear after passing clots, client may stay home.

Refer to MD   If client passing large, bright red clots or if unable to void

Emergency   Severe pain or if unable to void

Cross Reference   Blood in Urine; Urine, Dark-Colored

Etiology

Assessment

Treatment/ Teaching

Refer to MD

Emergency

Cross Reference   Abortion, Abruptio Placentae, Ectopic Pregnancy, Placenta Previa, Spotting

Hemorrhage from a dilated vein in the esophagus

Etiology   Esophageal veins become dilated in response to increased venous pressure caused by cirrhosis of the liver. Cirrhosis is usually caused by alcoholic liver disease.

Assessment   Usual symptoms include sudden weakness or fainting followed by hematemesis (90% of time) and melena. Pallor and shock may be present. Client may not be experiencing pain. History of alcohol abuse.

Treatment/ Teaching   Measures for shock until emergency aid arrives.

Refer to MD   Arrange for emergency transportation to hospital

Emergency   Arrange for emergency transportation to hospital

Cross Reference   Blood in Stools, Blood in Vomitus, Shock

BLOATING

Flatulent distention of the stomach

Etiology Retention of gas, medications, foods, excessive swallowing of air (e.g., gulping food or fluids); common problem following some surgical procedures

Assessment Determine if the client is able to pass flatus and stool, if there is excessive air swallowing (e.g., gum chewing), if there are any medications or ingested foods that may be the source of the problem. Assess history of any chronic illness (e.g., alcoholism or hypertension), pregnancy; if there are any ancillary symptoms (e.g., chest pain). R/o cardiac problem.

Treatment/ Teaching **If bloating related to retention of flatus:** Warm tub bath or heat to abdomen for 30 minutes. Restrict diet; avoid beans, cabbage, and other foods that may contribute to the problem. Sip 7-Up to help break up gas pockets or bubbles. Try antacids, especially those designed to break up gas (Digel, Mylanta II, Mylicon). Mild exercise (e.g., walking). Eat slowly. Avoid smoking. Avoid drinking hot beverages.

Refer to MD For evaluation of chronic problem and/or other serious ancillary symptoms

Emergency If cardiac distress present

Cross Reference Abdominal Pain, Chest Pain, Gas, Indigestion

BLOOD IN EYE (Subconjunctival Hemorrhage)

Bright red blood under the conjunctiva of the globe

Etiology   Trauma, Valsalva's maneuver, hard sustained sneezing or coughing, heavy lifting, blood dyscrasias

Assessment   Area of bleeding may be very small or may involve almost all the white of the eye around the cornea. Painless condition; noted only on visualization of eye.

Treatment/ Teaching   It is innocuous but alarms the client and observers. There is no effective treatment; it represents blood out of place (as does ecchymosis). Reassure client that gradual, spontaneous resolution will occur.

Refer to MD   If associated with trauma to eye, if bleeding covers the iris of the eye, or continuous pattern of increased/enlarging hemorrhage

Emergency

Cross Reference

Coughing up of blood

Etiology Recent vomiting or nosebleed, toxic inhalant, bronchopulmonary disease (e.g., bronchitis, tuberculosis, carcinoma, bronchiectasis), recent URI with cough, alcoholism, anticoagulant therapy

Assessment Bleeding of more than a few ounces is uncommon. Fatal hemorrhage is rare. When associated with chest pain and shock, hemoptysis suggests pulmonary infarction. Rely on history and ancillary symptoms. Determine color, approximate amount, history of similar episodes. (More than 1 tablespoon or so requires prompt attention.)

Treatment/ Teaching If associated with URI symptoms, cough meds (dextromethorphan-containing preparations) may be taken; moist air inhalations and fluids help.

Refer to MD For evaluation of nonemergency condition

Emergency If sudden onset and more than streaks or flecks of blood present; if associated with chest pain or shock

Cross Reference Bronchitis, Cough

Tarry stools or stools streaked with red blood

Etiology GI bleeding, hemorrhoids, rectal fissure or lesion, colitis, esophageal varices

Assessment Assess for history of GI bleeding (ulcers, colitis, esophageal varices), presence of abdominal pain, diarrhea, pain with passage of stool, history of hemorrhoids. Determine amount of bleeding. Rely on history and ancillary symptoms.

Treatment/ Teaching If minimal (less than 1 teaspoon) bright bleeding in formed stool, suspect hemorrhoids or rectal lesion. May try sitz bath.

Refer to MD For evaluation of any bleeding in formed stool, treatment of mild to moderate colitis, management of ulcer with mild to moderate abdominal pain unrelieved by home treatment

Emergency Moderate to large amounts of active rectal bleeding, tarry stools with GI symptoms, suspected esophageal varices, intractable pain

Cross Reference Black Stools; Bleeding from Esophageal Varices; Colitis; Constipation; Diarrhea; Food Poisoning; Gastroenteritis; Hemorrhoids; Rectal Bleeding; Salmonella Infection; Ulcer, Duodenal and Gastric

Presence of gross blood or microscopic red blood cells in urine

Etiology

Infections, trauma, glomerular disease, neoplasms, vascular accidents, anomalies, stones, coagulation defects

Assessment

When blood appears only during the **initial** period of voiding, the most likely source is the anterior urethra or prostate. When it appears during the **terminal** period of voiding, the most likely source is the posterior urethra, vesical neck or trigone. Blood **mixed in** with the total urine volume is from the kidneys, ureters, or bladder. Check for history of recent urinary tract procedure (e.g., post-TUR, urethral dilatation, catheterization). Determine presence of associated pain, frequency, urgency, hesitancy; whether urine is grossly bloody, dark in color, or if bleeding is occurring only during a certain portion of the stream; presence of fever. Coitus within past 24 hours is classic antecedent to hemorrhagic cystitis in females. Check if client is on anticoagulant therapy.

Treatment/ Teaching

Have client acidify urine by drinking cranberry juice. With recent TUR, dilatation, or catheterization: clear fluids (without caffeine) and recontact nurse if bleeding has not stopped in a few hours (needs to be seen quickly for hemorrhage).

Refer to MD

For evaluation and treatment of infection

Emergency

Gross bleeding and/or severe pain

Cross Reference

Bed Wetting (Peds); Bladder Pain; Bleeding After Urethral Dilatation; Burning on Urination; Kidney Stones; Prostatectomy, Post-op Care; Prostatitis; Urinary Tract Infection; Urine, Dark-Colored

Bright red bleeding or "coffee grounds" emesis

Etiology

Gastrointestinal bleeding (e.g., gastritis, gastric ulcer, esophageal varices)

Assessment

Check for history of sudden weakness or fainting, tarry stools, pallor, presence of shock, history of recent nosebleed or excessive coughing, presence of chest or abdominal pain. R/o recent ingestion of red-colored juice, Jell-o that would account for red coloration, history of alcoholism, steroids.

Treatment/ Teaching

Attempt to determine the amount of blood loss (e.g., 1 tsp or ½ cup or more). Save bloody emesis for testing by physician. Client may stay home if has 1 forceful emesis streaked with blood (especially if following a nosebleed or if has been coughing repeatedly or retching) and is otherwise asymptomatic.

Refer to MD

For evaluation if hematemesis recurs, but client's other symptoms are minimal

Emergency

If client has history of ulcers, esophageal varices, alcohol; if vomiting with bleeding occurs repeatedly; if amount of bleeding is increasing; if hematemesis is associated with melena

Cross Reference

Abdominal Pain; Black Stools; Bleeding from Esophageal Varices; Food Poisoning; Gastroenteritis; Tonsillectomy and Adenoidectomy, Post-op; Ulcer, Duodenal and Gastric

BLOOD UNDER THE NAIL (Subungual Hematoma)

Bleeding under a fingernail or toenail

Etiology Trauma (e.g., finger shut in door, finger or toe hit with a hammer)

Assessment R/o fracture.

Treatment/ Teaching Treatment best if carried out in first hour or less of the appearance of hematoma or injury, before the blood fibrin has set up. Puncture nail at darkest part or where hematoma has risen, using an extended paper clip heated to red or white hot in an open flame. Use only slight pressure since heat will burn hole in nail. Reheat paperclip prn. This is not a painful procedure and when blood is released, there is marked decrease in pain.

Refer to MD If unable to carry out procedure at home, if secondary infection or injury, increasing swelling and pain

Emergency

Cross Reference

An acute inflammatory conditon surrounding a hair follicle

Etiology   Staphylococcus aureus

Assessment   Rounded or conical; gradually enlarges then softens; opens spontaneously after a few days to 1 to 2 weeks, discharges core of necrotic tissue, pus.

Treatment/ Teaching   Warm soaks and/or compresses for 20 minutes, 4 times a day until lesion comes to a head and opens. If not opening, may need I&D, culture, antibiotics. Clean, dry dressing. Boil above lipline should be seen the same day because of possible cellulitis.

Refer to MD   For I&D and/or antibiotics, streaking, if infection and fever develop

Emergency

Cross Reference   Hot Pack (Glossary), Pimples

Food poisoning

Etiology

Ingestion of **Clostridium Botulinum**, found in canned, smoked, or vacuum-packed anaerobic foods, especially home-canned vegetables

Assessment

12 to 36 hours after ingestion of the toxin, visual disturbances (diplopia and loss of power of accommodation) appear. Other symptoms include dry throat and mouth, dysphagia, dysphonia, nausea and vomiting, prominent muscle weakness that impairs respirations. Sensorium remains clear, temperature normal. Progressive respiratory paralysis may lead to death without mechanical assistance.

Treatment/ Teaching

Bring sample of suspected food for testing. **Prevention:** Home-canned vegetables must be sterilized to destroy spores. Boiling any questionable food for 20 minutes can inactivate toxin, but punctured or swollen cans or jars with defective seals should be discarded.

Refer to MD

If suspicious food ingested, but minimal or no symptoms present

Emergency

Progressive symptoms present and/or respiratory distress

Cross Reference

Food Poisoning

Slow rate of heart contraction resulting in a slow pulse (heart rate slower than 60/minute)

Etiology   Increased vagal influence on the normal pacing mechanism of the heart. Common in athletes and young persons in vigorous health. May be due to meningitis, GI disturbances, pain, pressure on carotid sinus, eyeballs, or posterior pharynx, profuse hemorrhage. Found in clients convalescing from infectious diseases and in those with jaundice. May be the result of a faulty battery in an implanted pacemaker. Occurs commonly during rest or sleep.

Assessment   Uncomplicated sinus bradycardia produces no symptoms unless it is extreme, when it may lead to syncope and convulsions.

Treatment/ Teaching   Usually no treatment is required. Check for history of cardiac problems, possible pacemaker failure, heart block.

Refer to MD   For problems caused by underlying illness or infectious disease

Emergency   Fainting spells or decreased cerebration (i.e., weakness, confusion)

Cross Reference   Dysrhythmias

Vaginal bleeding that occurs when client is on oral contraceptives and at times other than the normal menstrual period

Etiology   Low levels of estrogen or progesterone

Assessment   Differentiate from regular menstrual period.

Treatment/ Teaching

If flow is light: Continue pills as usual and check with own MD.

If flow is moderate (needs to wear a pad): Double up on pills until bleeding stops, after which resume 1 pill a day for remainder of cycle unless bleeding recurs; notify MD.

If heavy flow without other symptoms: Have client take extra pill. If flow decreases, follow up with MD the following day. If heavy flow continues (more than 1 pad every 2 hours), client should be seen in emergency.

Refer to MD   For light or moderate flow as indicated above

Emergency   Hemorrhage (saturating more than 1 pad every 2 hours)

Cross Reference   Birth Control Pills, Spotting

Postpartum swelling, tenderness, and hardness of the breasts

Etiology   Retention of milk, vascular and lymphatic stasis, clogged milk duct

Assessment   Usual symptoms appear about third day postpartum and include swelling, hardness, tenderness of breast; slight fever may be present. R/o breast infection.

**Treatment/
Teaching**   **If breast-feeding:** Warm shower may help relieve initial engorgement. Encourage frequent breast-feedings. Massage breasts toward nipples, all quadrants. Supportive bra. Analgesics (acetaminophen or ASA). Manual expression of milk to alleviate extreme discomfort.

If not breast-feeding: Tight bra, ice packs, analgesics, no stimulants (e.g., shower).

Refer to MD If febrile; for meds to suppress lactation if not given after delivery

Emergency

**Cross
Reference**   Breast Infection, Ice Pack (Glossary)

Antibiotics the nursing mother should **NOT** take

Etiology

Assessment

Treatment/
Teaching

Drug	Potential Problem
Tetracycline	Staining of infant's teeth
Chloramphenicol	Blood dyscrasias
Flagyl (metronidazole)	Possible cancer in infant
Sulfonamides	Possible hemolytic anemia in infant
Nalidixic Acid	Possible hemolytic anemia in infant

Refer to MD

Emergency

Cross
Reference

BREAST INFECTION (Mastitis)

Inflammation of the breast

Etiology Usually staphylococcus; may be associated with clogged duct

Assessment Very common postpartum complication. Usual symptoms include flu-like syndrome with aching, malaise, muscle pain, fever (often 103° to 104°F), tender reddened area on 1 breast. A nipple fissure sometimes present. Check for sore, red, swollen area on breast. Check for red streaking on the breast tissue and axillary node swelling on affected side.

Treatment/ Teaching Hot packs to affected breast. If temp over 100°F, contact MD ASAP and discontinue nursing on affected breast. May self-express milk. If discharge from fissure or nipple present, stop breast-feeding. If previously diagnosed and mother is on tetracycline or chloramphenicol, breast-feeding **must** be discontinued.

Refer to MD To be seen same day for evaluation and antibiotic therapy

Emergency

Cross Reference Breast Engorgement, Breast-Feeding and Antibiotic Therapy, Fever, Hot Pack (Glossary)

Etiology

Assessment

Treatment/ Teaching

Refer to MD

Emergency

Cross Reference   Anaphylaxis; Asthma; Atelectasis; Bee Sting; Botulism; Chest Pain; Choking; Congestive Heart Failure; Convulsions; Cough; Diabetic Ketoacidosis; Electric Shock; Emphysema; Epiglottitis (Peds); Guillain-Barré Syndrome; Hyperventilation; Myocardial Infarction; Nose, Broken; Overdose; Pleurisy; Pneumonia; Pneumothorax; Pulmonary Edema; Pulmonary Embolus; Shock; Swallowing Difficulty

Etiology

Assessment

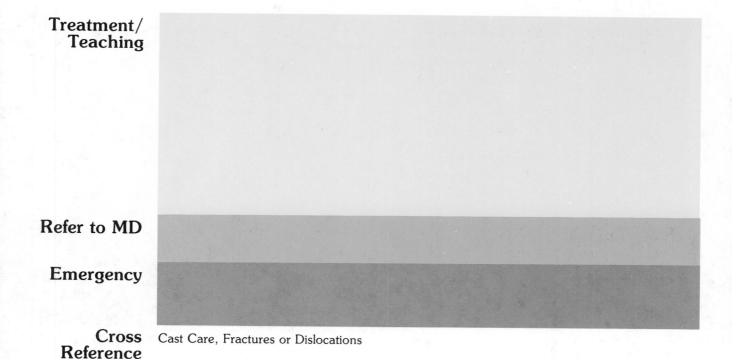

**Treatment/
Teaching**

Refer to MD

Emergency

**Cross
Reference**   Cast Care, Fractures or Dislocations

Inflammation of the bronchi

Etiology Viral or bacterial infections, chemical irritants, irritation

Assessment Common in viral infections, may follow the common cold. Early symptoms are those of URI (dry cough, nonproductive at first, progressing to more mucoid or mucopurulent secretions in more abundant amounts). Fever may occur for 3 to 5 days, following which acute symptoms subside. Cough may continue 2 to 3 weeks. R/o chronic bronchitis (symptoms usually not preceded by URI).

Treatment/ Teaching Bed rest. Clear fluids (8 ounce glass every hour) unless there is any cardiac contraindication. Vaporizer, steamy bathroom, or breathe steam from sink or bowl with towel over head. Expectorant and/or cough suppressant (e.g., Robitussin, Triaminic, 2/G). ASA for fever. Elevate head while in bed. Honey-lemon cough mix.

Refer to MD For evaluation and treatment

Emergency

Cross Reference Blood in Sputum, Cold Symptoms, Cough, Fever, Honey-Lemon Cough Mix (Glossary), Influenza, Upper Respiratory Infection

Bleeding into the tissue under unbroken skin

Etiology   Direct trauma to skin; secondary to blood disorders, anticoagulant therapy

Assessment   Rely on history and symptoms. Determine if client on anticoagulant therapy.

Treatment/ Teaching   Ice pack for 20 minute intervals several times daily for 1 to 2 days. Elevate area if possible. Protect area.

Refer to MD   For evaluation of large hematoma, if limb was compressed, evaluation of causes not related to trauma, symptoms of fracture

Emergency   Rapidly expanding, large hematoma unresponsive to ice and elevation at home

Cross Reference   Fractures or Dislocations, Hematoma, Ice Pack (Glossary)

Acute lateral angulation of the first metatarsophalangeal joint

Etiology   Usually shoes that push laterally on the great toe, congenital irregularities of first metatarsal

Assessment

Treatment/ Teaching   Keep pressure off bursa and toe with properly applied bunion pads (sometimes 2 are needed, 1 on top of the other). Can cut hole in shoe. Wear loosely fitting footwear. Avoid wearing shoes whenever possible.

Refer to MD   For treatment and/or evaluation of need for surgical intervention

Emergency

Cross Reference

Sensation of burning during voiding

Etiology   Infection of bladder or prostate, urethral irritation, nonspecific urethritis

Assessment   Check for presence of fever, back pain, frequency of urination, hesitancy, urgency, blood in the urine, penile discharge in men. Rely on history and ancillary symptoms.

Treatment/ Teaching   Fluids, especially cranberry juice. Avoid coffee, tea (they irritate bladder). Urinary analgesic prn. UA for culture and sensitivity (no antibiotic without culture first).

Refer to MD   For evaluation and treatment; be seen same day for gross hematuria, fever, severe discomfort

Emergency

Cross Reference   Bladder Pain; Bladder Trouble; Blood in Urine; Gonorrhea; Urinary Tract Infection; Urine, Dark-Colored

Injury due to chemicals, dry heat, electricity, flame, friction, radiation

Etiology   Thermal injury from flames, hot liquids or gases, chemicals, radiation

Assessment   Determine the cause, severity, extent, location of burned area. **First degree** produces erythema, **second degree** produces erythema and blistering, **third degree** produces full thickness skin loss, skin appears white in color and sloughs off. No pain evident with third degree burn. Determine presence of shock, cardiac and respiratory distress. Use "rule of nines" in estimating percentage of body burned: head and neck equals 9%, entire arm each 9%, anterior and posterior surfaces of upper trunk each 9%, anterior and posterior of lower trunk each 9%, anterior and posterior surfaces of legs each 9%.

Treatment/ Teaching   **First degree thermal**: Cold packs (not ice) to area. ASA every 4 hours prn. Do not use ointment that leaves an oily film (e.g., Vaseline). May use Noxema. Keep area clean. Cover with clean, dry dressing. Watch for infection.
Chemical burn: Wash off chemical, use cold compresses.

Refer to MD   For second degree burn, if burn infected

Emergency   Any third degree, large area second degree, radiation, or electric burn. Arrange emergency transportation to hospital if shock, respiratory or cardiac distress are present.

Cross Reference   Electric Shock, Shock, Wound Infection

Inflammation of a bursa (fibrous sac lined with synovial membrane containing a small quantity of synovial fluid)

Etiology   Friction, trauma, no obvious cause

Assessment   Bursae are found between tendon and bone, skin and bone, and muscle and muscle. Usual symptoms include pain, swelling, tenderness, limitation of motion in the associated joint or joints. Recovery is usually in 1 to 2 weeks, if acute. Attacks often simulate arthritis. Condition may be acute or chronic. Acute symptoms may follow unusual exercise or effort.

Treatment/ Teaching   Rest the affected extremity until pain and muscle spasms subside. Analgesics. Local heat. Following a cortisone injection, pain may be more severe for 24 hours. Use heat to the injection site to speed up absorption of drug and for comfort. Client may need codeine or other narcotic initially to manage pain.

Refer to MD   For evaluation and for management of pain

Emergency

Cross Reference   Arthritis

Pain, tenderness in the muscle area of the calf

Etiology   Injury, thrombophlebitis, potassium depletion, pregnancy, varicose veins

Assessment   Rely on history and ancillary symptoms. Check onset, location, character, intensity, history of similar pain, radiation, things that relieve or exacerbate it. To R/o tendon injury, check if client can stand on his tiptoes; check for problems with circulation in leg, check pedal pulse. R/o fracture, tendon injury, soft-tissue injury.

Treatment/ Teaching   **Thrombophlebitis:** See cross reference card.

Injury: Ice packs, elevation.

Pregnancy: See cross reference card.

Potassium deficiency (due to diuretics): Increase intake of bananas, orange juice, cantaloupe, meats.

Refer to MD   For evaluation of fracture or injury, management of hypokalemia or thrombophlebitis

Emergency   Circulatory impairment in leg, severe injury, or increasing swelling and pain

Cross Reference   Fractures or Dislocations; Pregnancy, Minor Discomforts Of; Strain; Thrombophlebitis; Varicose Veins

CANKER SORE (Aphthous Stomatitis)

Shallow, mucosal ulcer in mouth

Etiology Acidic foods, stress situations, unknown causes

Assessment Ulcer is flat with fairly even borders surrounded by erythema; frequently painful; often covered by a pseudomembrane, not vesicular like herpes. Canker sore tends to be a single lesion on floor of mouth; herpes tends to be multiple and on tongue as well as on other surfaces.

Treatment/ Teaching Fluids. Soft diet. Dip Q-Tip in baking soda and apply to lesion prior to meal (decreases pain and aids oral intake). Saline rinses and gargles. Gly-Oxide or Camphophenique to lesion; Orabase also helpful.

Refer to MD If no healing in 1 to 3 weeks; if secondary infection or stomatitis develops

Emergency

Cross Reference Cold Sore; Herpes Simplex

Guidelines for care of problems with a cast

Etiology

Assessment Rely on history and ancillary symptoms. Determine how old the cast is and reason for its placement. If a new cast, assess for poor circulation.

Treatment/ Teaching

Drying: If cast becomes wet, towel it off and and blow dry with a portable hair dryer.

Cracking: Bind with wide adhesive tape to secure; tell client to return to doctor for repair during normal office hours.

Pain & Swelling: Check circulation; elevate above level of the heart; call back in 20 to 30 minutes if not relieved.

Cleaning: Apply white shoe polish.

Itching: Do not stick anything inside the cast. Coat hangers and other long pointed objects can abrade the skin and predispose to infection. A light dusting of talc or directing a hair blower, **set on cool**, into the cast may be helpful.

Circulation: Check for evidence of tight cast (throbbing pain not relieved by elevation above the level of the heart; cold, cyanotic, or poorly blanching digits). Refer client to MD.

Bleeding: Draw a circle around the discolored area at its border, apply an ice pack. Refer client to MD.

Refer to MD For cast repair or problems with circulation or bleeding

Emergency

Cross Reference Fractures or Dislocations, Numbness

A diffuse inflammation of connective tissue or skin

Etiology   Usually B-hemolytic strep or staphylococcus

Assessment   Fever, chills, malaise, and headache may be present. Area involved is usually red, swollen, painful, warm, with poorly defined borders. R/o erysipelas.

Treatment/   Rest involved part, elevate when possible. Local application of moist hot packs, especially
Teaching   towels under a plastic wrap (Saran Wrap, plastic bag). Check for current tetanus immunization, especially if initial lesion is a wound. To assess the degree of progression of the infection, draw a line at the border of the redness. Use line as a guide to determine spread of infection.

Refer to MD   For diagnosis and antibiotic therapy; cellulitis on the face needs to be seen same day

Emergency   Massive and extensive infection, or infection is spreading rapidly

Cross   Bee Sting, Facial Pain, Fever, Hot Pack (Glossary), Wound Infection
Reference

Etiology

Assessment

Treatment/ Teaching

Refer to MD

Emergency

Cross Reference   Stroke

A cyst on the edge of the eyelid, resulting from retained secretion of the meibomian gland

Etiology   Unknown

Assessment   Usually appears as a painless, unsightly bump in the substance of the eyelid; no threat to vision. Very infrequently it may become infected and develop into a purulent abscess. R/o sty.

Treatment/ Teaching   Chalazions are ordinarily left alone unless they become unsightly or repeatedly infected. Warm compresses may help accelerate resolution during initial development (usually will be of no benefit after cyst is firmly established).

Refer to MD   For treatment of infection and/or surgical removal

Emergency

Cross Reference   Sty in Eye

Advice for clients on chemotherapy

Etiology

Assessment

Drug, number of days postadministration; disease status; disease entity, newness, severity; duration of symptoms (can include nausea, vomiting, fatigue, hair loss, menstrual irregularities, decreased immunity [from low white count], and bleeding tendency [from low platelet count]). Prescribed antiemetics can have extrapyramidal side effects. Refer to PDR for individual drug considerations.

Treatment/ Teaching

For clients on chemotherapy, the 10 to 14 days or 2 weeks after treatment is usually the most critical time. This is when the blood count is low and client may develop secondary infections that can worsen rapidly. All clients who are febrile or feeling ill and fit this situation need to be seen quickly.

Nausea and vomiting: Bland, dry, bulky foods; fluids; antiemetics as ordered (may need suppository form); progressive diet as tolerated. Can easily become dehydrated if not controlled.

Fatigue: Rest, good nutrition. Often a sign of low WBC.

Decreased immunity: Stay out of crowds and away from persons with colds, flu, or contagious disease. Take temperature every 4 hours while awake; report any elevation above 100°F immediately.

Bleeding tendency: Observe carefully for signs of hemorrhage (hematuria, bruising, bleeding gums, nosebleeds etc.) or shock. Report any signs of bleeding to MD.

Hair loss: Reassure that hair will grow back when therapy is discontinued. Short haircut; buy wig/scarves/hat.

Menstrual irregularities: Reassure that menses usually return to normal after therapy is discontinued. Offer guidance regarding menopausal symptoms prn. Continue use of nonhormonal birth control.

Refer to MD

If febrile, for cold/flu symptoms, increased tendency to bleed, intractable vomiting, evidence of dehydration

Emergency

Cross Reference

Dehydration, Nausea and Vomiting, Menopausal Syndrome

Discomfort or pain in the thoracic region

Etiology
Cardiac: Angina, myocardial infarction, myopericarditis, pericardial effusion or tamponade, aortic dissection or aneurysm, pulmonary embolism or infarction

Noncardiac: Arthritis of upper spine, cardiac neurosis, emotional disorders, hiatus hernia, acute or chronic cholecystitis, acute pancreatitis, cardiospasm, peptic ulcer, esophageal pain, costochondritis, strain or inflammation of pectoral and intercostal muscles and ligaments, post-myocardial infarction syndrome, periarthritis of left shoulder, spontaneous pneumothorax, pleurisy, spinal-cord disease, mediastinal tumor, emphysema

Assessment
Rely on history and ancillary symptoms. Carefully evaluate quality of pain, its location, radiation, duration, and the factors that precipitate, aggravate, or relieve it. Localized pain, increased by deep inspiration and relieved by heat, rest, and mild analgesics without cardiac history is characteristic of **chest wall pain. Cardiac pain** is persistent, steadily increasing, and accompanied by radiation (to neck, arms, jaw), SOB, diaphoresis, cyanosis, weakness, and nausea/vomiting.

Treatment/ Teaching
Chest wall or pleuritic pain: ASA, heat to chest.

Cardiac pain: Arrange for transportation to hospital. Home treatment is not appropriate.

Refer to MD
If pain seems to be of noncardiac nature, is not severe, if unaccompanied by other serious ancillary symptoms

Emergency
Severe pain, cardiac and/or respiratory distress

Cross Reference
Aneurysm; Angina; Anxiety; Atelectasis; Bloating; Costochondritis; Fatigue; Gall Bladder Colic; Hiatus Hernia; Myocardial Infarction; Pleurisy; Pneumothorax; Pulmonary Edema; Pulmonary Embolus; Ulcer, Duodenal and Gastric; Upper Respiratory Infection

Etiology

Assessment

Treatment/ Teaching

Refer to MD

Emergency

Cross Reference Chickenpox (Peds)

Etiology

Assessment

**Treatment/
Teaching**

Refer to MD

Emergency

**Cross
Reference**   Fever, Shakiness

Symptom caused by an obstruction blocking the airway

Etiology Foreign body in throat

Assessment Client's inability to talk is indicative of a foreign body aspiration. The universal sign of distress is that of the client grasping at his throat.

Treatment/ Teaching Ask the caller if the choking person can talk or cough. **If yes**: Watch person carefully and reassure. **If not***: Instruct the caller (rescuer) as follows: stand behind the client, lean the client forward, and support the client's chest with 1 arm (bringing arm underneath the client's arm and placing hand flat against the client's opposite shoulder). With free hand, give 4, quick, upward, glancing blows to the client's posterior thoracic area. If this does not dislodge the foreign body, make a fist with 1 hand (tucking the thumb under the fingers) and with both arms, encircle the client under the arms at the level of the lower sternum. Standing behind the client, with the enclosed fist next to the client's sternum, give 1 or 2 sharp thrusts inward. If the choking person is alone, s/he can lean over a chair and give a blow to the sternum. Continue until foreign body is dislodged.

Children: Try to clear airway by putting child in an upside-down position and thump on child's back. Arrange for emergency aid as needed.

For fish bones stuck in the throat: Eat bread and drink milk. If scratchy throat persists over 2 hours, come to ER.

For small piece of meat stuck in the throat and partially obstructing the airway: Dissolve 1 teaspoon meat tenderizer in 8 ounces water. Sip and gargle solution until meat can be dislodged.

*If person calling does not know rescue technique already, arrange for emergency aid first and then instruct person to attempt to dislodge foreign body.

Refer to MD If aspirated foreign body may be lodged in lungs and if respiratory distress is minimal or absent

Emergency Severe respiratory distress, unable to dislodge foreign body, unconsciousness

Cross Reference Cyanosis, Drooling, Meat-Tenderizer Solution (Glossary), Pneumonia, Wheezing, Swallowing Difficulty

Vesicular eruption on skin or mucous membranes of mouth

Etiology   Herpes simplex virus

Assessment   Recurrent, small, grouped vesicles on an erythematous base around or in mouth. May follow minor infections, trauma, stress, sun exposure. Can recur in the same location for years. R/o herpes zoster, impetigo, canker sore. Herpes type 1 (simplex) is usually more painful to touch than impetigo and may also appear as multiple vesicular lesions on tongue and other surfaces of the mouth; canker sore is usually a single lesion on floor of mouth.

Treatment/ Teaching   **Lesions outside mouth:** Fluids (especially cold fluids), ice chips, popsicles. Cold compresses to external cold sore. Gly-Oxide or Camphophenique to single lesion. Bland diet.

Multiple lesions in mouth: Cold fluids. Soft, bland diet. Glyoxide to lesions. Benadryl-Maalox mouthwash as needed for discomfort (½ Benadryl and ½ Maalox). Caution client to avoid touching the lesion to reduce the chance of infecting another area of the body or another individual.

Refer to MD   For evaluation and treatment of multiple lesions in mouth or on face, or difficulty swallowing

Emergency

Cross Reference   Canker Sore; Herpes Simplex; Impetigo; Lip Lesions

Signs and symptoms of the common cold

Etiology Viral

Assessment Usual symptoms include malaise, fever, sore throat, nasal discomfort with watery discharge followed shortly by mucoid to purulent discharge and nasal congestion, headache, cough. Incubation period is short, usually 18 to 48 hours. Onset is abrupt. Ask if any family members or day care playmates are ill. School-age children usually bring viral infections home; adults are more likely to bring bacterial infections home.

Treatment/ Teaching ASA prn fever and aches (If client less than 15 years of age, or on anticoagulant drugs or chronic GI problems recommend acetaminophen). Rest. Decongestants (e.g., Sudafed, CTM). Expectorants (e.g., Robitussin, 2/G) prn cough. Clear fluids. Saline nose drops. Vaporizer. Honey-lemon cough mixture. No dairy products. Watch for persistent fever, green or yellow purulent sputum or drainage from nose, ear pain, chest pain, dyspnea, persistent sore throat.

Refer to MD For treatment and evaluation of secondary infection

Emergency

Cross Reference Bronchitis, Cough, Ear Infection, Fever, Honey-Lemon Cough Mix (Glossary), Nasal Congestion, Pleurisy, Pneumonia, Saline Nose Drops (Glossary), Sinus Congestion, Sinus Infection, Sore Throat, Upper Respiratory Infection

A chronic, nonspecific, inflammatory, and ulcerative disease of the colon

Etiology   Unknown, often related to stress

Assessment Primarily a disease of adolescents and young adults, but may have onset in any age group. Usual symptoms include bloody diarrhea with lower abdominal cramps, mild abdominal tenderness, weight loss, and fever. Diarrhea stools may number 30 to 40 a day with blood and mucus in the stool (a chief manifestation) or passage of blood and mucus alone.

Treatment/ Teaching No milk products; low-fiber diet, minimal sugar and spices. Clear fluids (e.g., Gatorade, 7-Up, ginger ale, water). Heat to abdomen prn cramping.

Refer to MD For mild to moderate symptoms

Emergency   Frequent bloody stools accompanied by fever, intractable pain, or dehydration

Cross Reference Abdominal Pain, Blood in Stools, Diarrhea, Giardiasis, Rectal Bleeding, Salmonella Infection

Complete loss of consciousness

Etiology

Intracranial: Head injuries, CVA, CNS infections, tumors, convulsive disorders, degenerative diseases, increased intracranial pressure

Extracranial: Vascular (shock or hemorrhage), myocardial infarction, metabolic (e.g., diabetic acidosis), uremia, hypoglycemia, electrolyte imbalance; intoxication (drugs, metals, gases, alcohol); miscellaneous (e.g., hyperthermia, hypothermia, electric shock, anaphylaxis, severe systemic infections)

Assessment

Rely on history and ancillary symptoms. Interrogate client if initially lucid or rely on client's family, friends, or attendants. Inquire specifically about client's occupation; previous mental, emotional, or physical illness; trauma; epilepsy; hypertension; use of alcohol and drugs.

Treatment/ Teaching

Emergency: Keep airway open. Place client on side with head well extended. CPR and treatment for shock prn.

Not an emergency: May be expected outcome for terminally ill client; may be cared for at home. Check on arrangements for home nursing care.

Refer to MD

If coma is expected, if help is needed with home care

Emergency

Sudden onset, need to maintain life-support systems

Cross Reference

Anaphylaxis; Convulsions; Diabetic Ketoacidosis; Electric Shock; Head Injury; Hypoglycemia; Myocardial Infarction; Overdose, Drug; Shock; Stroke

Mental state of being out of touch with reality; associated with a clouding of consciousness

Etiology   Seizure disorder, CVA, trauma, chronic brain syndrome, alcohol ingestion, head injury, senile dementia, medications, psychosis, diabetes, exposure to toxic chemicals

Assessment   Rely on history and ancillary symptoms. Determine degree of client's orientation, i.e., does he know his name? where he is? date? (i.e., "oriented x 3").

Treatment/ Teaching   Try to put client in most familiar surroundings. Keep area well lit. Do not leave alone; have client watched by someone familiar to him.

Refer to MD   For evaluation of acute problem or associated symptoms, management of a chronic problem; refer to psychiatrist prn psychotic disorder

Emergency

Cross Reference   Convulsions, Hallucinations, Head Injury, Psychosis, Stroke

Etiology

Assessment

**Treatment/
Teaching**

Refer to MD

Emergency

**Cross
Reference**   Allergies, Bronchitis, Cold Symptoms, Congestive Heart Failure, Emphysema, Hay Fever, Nasal Congestion, Pneumonia, Pulmonary Edema, Sinus Congestion, Sinus Infection, Upper Respiratory Infection

Failure of the heart to maintain an adequate output, resulting in congestion in the pulmonary and/or systemic circulation and diminished blood flow to the tissues.

Etiology

Most common cause in US is ischemic heart disease secondary to coronary artery disease, hypertension, or arteriosclerotic heart disease. Other common causes are valvular disease and congenital heart disease.

Assessment

Gradual or sudden onset of symptoms that include loss of energy, fatigue, weakness, dyspnea, pedal edema, cyanosis, mental confusion, impairment of memory, loss of concentration, orthopnea, paroxysmal nocturnal dyspnea, weight gain over past 2 days (fluid retention). Review if correct medication dosages, diet, and activity procedures are being followed. Assess if this is a chronic or acute condition.

Treatment/ Teaching

Bed rest in semi-Fowler's position (or sit in chair) if symptoms are chronic and not increasing.

Refer to MD

If distress is gradually increasing

Emergency

If respiratory distress is severe or of sudden onset

Cross Reference

Cough, Dysrhythmias, Nausea and Vomiting, Pulmonary Edema

Inflammation of the transparent membrane that lines the inner surface of the eyelids and reflects over the surface of the eyeball

Etiology Bacterial or viral

Assessment Usual symptoms include redness, itching, burning of the eye. If there is a purulent discharge and considerable crusting of the eyelashes, the origin is usually bacterial. If the discharge is more serous, the origin may be viral. No actual pain or loss of vision; minimal light sensitivity. Many bacterial and viral forms of conjunctivitis are contagious. Condition commonly accompanies a URI.

Treatment/ Teaching Avoid rubbing eye, infection may be contagious. Apply cool compresses to eyes periodically for 24 hours. Bathe eyes with warm water to remove discharge or crusting (use separate cotton ball for each eye). Use separate towels from others in home.

Refer to MD For treatment of symptoms not responding to home treatment

Emergency

Cross Reference Eye, Itching; Eyes, Bloodshot; Iritis; Upper Respiratory Infection

Infrequent and often difficult evacuation of hard, dry feces

Etiology   Diet; physical inactivity or prolonged bed rest; organic and functional causes; drugs, e.g., codeine or other narcotic analgesics

Assessment   Consider client constipated only if defecation is unexplainably delayed for a matter of days, or if the stools are unusually hard, dry, and difficult to pass. Suspect organic causes when there are sudden, unexplained changes in bowel habits or blood in the stool. Check drug and usual food intake.

**Treatment/
Teaching**   Establish regular evacuation time. Diet may need to be increased in 1) food intake; 2) fiber content (bran, raw fruits, and vegetables); 3) fluid intake (6 to 8 glasses of fluid per day and 1 glass hot water with lemon juice before breakfast). Moderate physical exercise. Laxative if indicated (e.g., Metamucil, Milk of Magnesia). Enema, especially oil retention, if indicated and client has had no recent bowel surgery. Glycerine suppository.

Refer to MD   For evaluation and treatment of chronic problem; if onset is sudden and unexplained

Emergency   Vomiting, abdominal distention, fever, significant rectal or lower GI bleeding

**Cross
Reference**   Abdominal Pain; Blood in Stools; Pregnancy, Minor Discomforts Of; Rectal Bleeding

Etiology

Assessment

Treatment/ Teaching

Refer to MD

Emergency

Cross Reference   Corneal Abrasions, Eye Pain

Paroxysmal disorders of cerebral function

Etiology   Hyperpyrexia, CNS infections, parasitic infections, metabolic disturbances, convulsive or toxic agents or poisons, cerebral hypoxia, expanding brain lesions, brain defects, cerebral edema, cerebral trauma, anaphylaxis, cerebral infarct or hemorrhage, withdrawal from drugs or alcohol

Assessment   Sudden in onset and of brief duration; characterized by recurrent attacks involving changes in the state of consciousness, motor activity, or sensory phenomena. Classification of seizures: Grand mal (major epilepsy), petit mal (minor epilepsy), Jacksonian epilepsy, psychomotor seizures, status epilepticus, febrile convulsions, massive spasms.

Syncope: Differs from seizures in that the muscles are flaccid, there are no convulsive movements initially, and the attack subsides with increased brain blood flow in recumbency.

In hysteria: There is usually no loss of consciousness, incontinence, tongue biting, or self-injury; client may be resistive and the convulsion erratic and atypical.

Treatment/ Teaching   Protect client from injury during the seizure. Remove any furniture or objects that client might harm self on. Do not forceably insert anything in mouth. Observe kinds of movement the client makes, which parts of the body are affected, and the approximate length of the seizure. Evaluate need for transportation to medical facility by car or by ambulance if client appears stable. Postictal state normally lasts from a few minutes to several hours; after a grand mal seizure, the client cannot be aroused, then begins by degrees to regain consciousness and finally awakens (sometimes alert, but often confused, suffering from headache, malaise, nausea). Clients with known seizure disorder need not come in after a seizure unless advised by MD to do so or if complications occur. Check if client with known seizure disorder has neglected to take prescribed medicine.

Refer to MD   If client has no history of seizures, for evaluation of client's status and need to alter anticonvulsant meds

Emergency   Repetitive seizures, loss of consciousness, severe respiratory distress

Cross Reference   Anaphylaxis, Balance Problems, Coma, Confusion, Cyanosis, Drowsiness, Fever, Head Injury, Heat Stroke, Hypoglycemia, Meningitis

CORNEAL ABRASION

A scratch on the cornea, which usually removes the outer epithelial layer

Etiology

Irritation to cornea caused by prolonged wearing of **hard** contact lenses, foreign body, or other trauma

Assessment

Symptoms usually occur immediately with trauma but can be delayed several hours with contact lens irritation or a foreign body and consist of extreme pain, excess watering of the eye, sensitivity to light; iritis usually absent.

Treatment/ Teaching

Lie in darkened room with eyes closed. Cold compresses or ice packs to reduce swelling. Condition is usually self-healing, but may require some eye drops and analgesic for pain management or removal of foreign body. To reduce discomfort, securely attach an eye patch over the affected eye. If client wears contact lens, s/he may begin limited wearing of them after several days of being asymptomatic.

Refer to MD

For management of pain, for removal of foreign body, for evaluation of purulent drainage or any symptoms that persist longer than 24 hours

Emergency

Alteration of vision, severe pain, or penetrating trauma

Cross Reference

Eye Pain

Inflammation of the cartilage at point where the rib joins the sternum

Etiology Unknown; sometimes associated with history of injury

Assessment Localized tenderness and ill-defined pain with or without localized swelling at 1 or more costochondral or chondrosternal junctions; commonly affects upper ribs; pain may be intensified by deep breathing and movement of trunk; a common cause of chest-wall pain.

Treatment/ Teaching Heat to affected area. Analgesics. Reassurance.

Refer to MD For management of pain if no relief with mild analgesics or if cardiac symptoms present

Emergency

Cross Reference Chest Pain

Sudden expulsion of air from the lungs, accompanied by an explosive noise made by opening the glottis

Etiology   Acute or chronic respiratory disease, congestive heart failure, otitis media, irritation (e.g., due to smoking, presence of foreign body)

Assessment   Check for history of recent URI versus chronic illness, if cough is dry or productive, characteristics of sputum; presence or absence of fever, chest pain, shortness of breath, wheezing, cyanosis, excessive perspiring, night sweats, history of recent exposure to person with communicable disease.

Treatment/ Teaching   **Acute, virally induced:** Clear fluids. Expectorant (e.g., 2/G, Robitussin) to help raise secretions. Vaporizer. Elevate head when sleeping. Honey-lemon cough mixture. Throat lozenges or cough drops prn.

Refer to MD   For treatment of bacterial infection, evaluation of chronic or persistent cough with or without fever, mild chest pain, wheezing (without severe dyspnea)

Emergency   Severe chest pain, severe dyspnea or cyanosis, wheezing with severe dyspnea, or blood in sputum

Cross Reference   Asthma, Blood in Sputum, Bronchitis, Cold Symptoms, Congestive Heart Failure, Emphysema, Honey-Lemon Cough Mix (Glossary), Pneumonia, Upper Respiratory Infection, Wheezing

Sudden painful contraction of skeletal muscles

Etiology   Strenuous exercise, positional cause, chronic illness, medications, trauma, phlebitis

Assessment   Rely on history and ancillary symptoms. Check for pedal pulse.

**Treatment/
Teaching**   Moist heat or ice pack prn discomfort. ASA. Gentle massage, if related to positional cause or exercise.

Refer to MD   For evaluation if recurring problem, suspected thrombophlebitis, occlusive artery disease of leg or foot, or if medication is cause

Emergency   Evidence of dramatically decreased circulation to limb

**Cross
Reference**   Hot Pack and Ice Pack (Glossary), Strain, Thrombophlebitis

Hypoxic tissue manifested by a bluish tinge

Etiology Respiratory problems (i.e., chronic COPD, CHF, emphysema), croup/epiglottitis, asthma, breath holding (peds), temper tantrum (peds), foreign-body aspiration, seizures, drug overdose, atelectasis, pneumothorax, cardiac problems

Assessment Rely on history and ancillary symptoms.

Treatment/ Teaching
For foreign body aspiration: see cross reference "Choking".
Home treatment with oxygen: see cross references "Emphysema," "Oxygen Information."

Refer to MD As needed for management of chronic problem

Emergency Onset of sudden, acute respiratory distress

Cross Reference Asthma, Atelectasis, Choking, Convulsions, Emphysema, Myocardial Infarction, Oxygen Information, Pneumothorax, Poisoning, Pulmonary Embolus

Guidelines to follow in handling situations involving death

Etiology

Assessment

Treatment/ Teaching

Often the Medical Examiner will request a call to the attending MD to determine if the physician will sign the death certificate.

Types of deaths requiring investigation by the Medical Examiner: Violence (homicide, suicide—immediate or delayed); sudden, unexpected death (no direct MD knowledge, not seen by MD in last 36 hours, no treatment in 2 weeks); poisoning (food or chemical); industrial (on-the-job); death from surgery; drug overdose, self-induced; deaths in custody (jail or mental institution); solitary deaths (private residence); death of unidentified person or persons without adequate identification (e.g., airplane crash); death in emergency room, when MD cannot certify a death by natural causes.

Types of deaths usually NOT requiring investigation by the Medical Examiner: Client seen by MD in past 24 hours, expected death. In the latter case, you may need to notify MD or assist family by calling funeral home, offering support, etc.

Medical Examiner 24-hour phone: _____
                                            (write in)

Fill in protocol specific to your agency or county.

Refer to MD

Emergency

Cross Reference

Loss of body fluid (fluid intake is inadequate to replace fluid output)

Etiology Inadequate fluid intake, intractable vomiting or diarrhea, electrolyte imbalance, fever, heat prostration

Assessment Most visible signs are decreased urinary output (urinating less than every 8 hours or urinating small amounts), decreased fluid intake, decreased skin turgor and shrunken, corregated tongue. Lethargy, weakness, confusion, and shock may also by present. Check fluid intake and output (urine, stool, emesis, perspiration). To check skin turgor, have observer pinch and raise skin on client's forearm. If well hydrated, the skin should have elastic quality and fall back into place. If inadequate hydration, skin will form a "tent" and not show elastic quality. Check for chronic illness such as diabetes, if client on Coumadin, chemotherapy, or other meds that might affect the heart or the electrolyte balance.

Treatment/ Teaching Fluids, if client is not vomiting (Gatorade especially good because of electrolyte content); tepid bath and ASA or acetaminophen if febrile.

Refer to MD If urinary output inadequate or other dehydration signs present; for antiemetics

Emergency Shock or apparent cardiac involvement, unconsciousness

Cross Reference Anorexia; Chemotherapy; Diarrhea; Fever; Food Poisoning; Gastroenteritis; Giardiasis; Heat Prostration; Kidney Stones; Nausea and Vomiting; Salmonella Infection; Urine, Dark-Colored

Abnormal mental condition characterized by hallucinations or illusions

Etiology Fever, drugs, emotional disorder, DTs (alcoholism)

Assessment Clouding of consciousness with impaired thinking, memory, perception, attention, and reality testing. Client may show vagueness, uncertainty, hesitancy in speech, minor errors in thinking; may be confused with slow responses and impaired orientation, loss of motor-control skills, incoherent speech, delusions, and hallucinations.

Treatment/ Teaching Depends on source and extent of problem. Refer for mental health counseling prn for evaluation of psychologic functioning or alcoholism.

Refer to MD For diagnosis and treatment if drug-related, if associated with fever, or if client acutely ill

Emergency If client is out of control and/or potentially dangerous

Cross Reference Fever, Hallucinations, Psychosis

Abscess, trauma, bleeding, or pain requiring intervention when private dentist is not reachable

Etiology Pain following dental extraction or procedure; trauma; infection

Assessment Check for facial or jaw pain and swelling, fever, or unpleasant taste in mouth, to help differentiate abscess. Check on recent dental history.

Treatment/ Teaching **Pain:** Analgesic (may need order from on-call MD) prn pain. Ice pack or heat prn discomfort.

Abscess: Be seen for appropriate Rx (antibiotic, pain med; cardiac client may need prophylactic penicillin before dental procedure).

Bleeding: Have client roll up a small piece of gauze and bite down on bleeding area.

Refer to MD (dentist) If abscess or gingival infection suspected; if bleeding not controlled

Emergency Traumatic tooth avulsion (Emergency Dentist _____)
                                                    Telephone Number

Cross Reference Tooth Avulsion

A mental state characterized by sadness and lowered self-esteem

Etiology   Reaction to a life event, anger turned inwards, means of controlling other people, endogenous

Assessment   Symptoms include lowered mood (varies in intensity from sadness to hopelessness), difficulty in thinking (trouble concentrating), loss of interest, negative self-concept, delusional ideas (hypochondriacal, self-accusatory, or persecutory), depersonalization (feelings of unreality), disturbance in sleep, loss of appetite, weight loss or gain, constipation, reduced sexual desire and potency, loss of energy, disturbance of menstrual function, and various other somatic complaints. Determine how long client has felt this way, if there are changes of interest in previously enjoyed activities.

Is there any thought of harming self or committing suicide? If so, is there a plan? Are means available? Have past attempts been made? If so, how? Were they treated medically? Inquire about any recent, major life events (e.g., death, marriage, new child, divorce, illness, etc.).

Treatment/ Teaching   If symptoms are minimal, help client look at alternatives (e.g., change activities, be with supportive friends, increase exercise, balance diet, etc.). Recognize that depression is a normal reaction to some life events. Encourage client to call back next day (if appropriate) or follow-up with MD.

Refer to MD   For mental health counseling if client responds in the affirmative to several of the above questions; if client currently in therapy, contact the therapist or consult with psychiatric resource person

Emergency   Obtain help immediately if client is suicidal, has a definite plan, and means are available. Fill in procedure for your facility here:

Cross Reference   Fatigue, Lethargy, Postpartum Depression, Suicide

Inflammation of the skin

Etiology Direct skin contact with offending plants, chemicals, or other irritants

Assessment Rash often on exposed parts or in bizarre, asymmetric patterns; pattern of eruption may be diagnostic (e.g., linear for plants that have been brushed by client). Check for history of contact to allergens (e.g., chemicals or irritants, poison ivy, soaps, lotions, or other skin agents).

Treatment/ Teaching Wash affected area (if contact with poison or chemical). Cool compresses. May use antihistamine (e.g., CTM, Benadryl) or Calamine to control itching.

Refer to MD If skin is burned due to exposure to chemical; if symptoms not managed with home care or complications develop; for wheezing or swelling of eyes, mouth, genitalia

Emergency Severe allergic reaction

Cross Reference Athlete's Foot, Genitalia Problems (Peds), Nettles Contact, Poison Ivy or Oak, Scabies

Syndrome characterized by disordered metabolism and hyperglycemia due to an absolute deficiency of insulin secretion or reduction in its biologic effectiveness

Etiology   Common denominator of those destined to become diabetic is genetic predisposition. Other factors include obesity, physical and emotional stress, pregnancy, viral infections, autoimmunity, current medications, pancreatitis, possibly the excessive ingestion of refined sugars.

Assessment   Classic symptoms are polyuria, polydipsia, polyphagia with weight loss, recurrent blurred vision, and fatigue.

Treatment/   Moderate exercise is a good means of utilizing fat and carbohydrates for diabetic clients. Rein-
Teaching   force adherence to diet and insulin therapy, need for client to know how to test urine for sugar and acetone, need for careful personal hygiene, especially with regard to feet, skin, and teeth. Prompt medical attention to surface injuries that are not healing properly with appropriate first-aid treatment.

Refer to MD   For diagnosis, for complications of diabetes, or for unrelated illness or trauma

Emergency   Ketoacidosis

Cross   Diabetic Ketoacidosis; Diabetic Persons with Illness; Insulin Reaction; Thirst, Excessive; Urine,
Reference   Excessive Output

Diabetic hyperglycemia with spilling of ketones into the urine

Etiology Insufficient insulin, failure to take insulin, febrile illnesses or illnesses causing vomiting and/or diarrhea

Assessment Onset is gradual (usually days before client appears ill). Client may complain of extreme thirst; skin is dry and often flushed; respirations are exaggerated, deep, and fast; breath may smell of acetone (fruity odor); pulse may be weak and rapid. Increasing lethargy may progress to comatose state.

Treatment/ Teaching Rely on history and ancillary symptoms. Check insulin requirements and usage. Check urine for sugar and acetone.

Refer to MD If client is alert and urine shows large amount of sugar or any acetone; for treatment of concurrent illness

Emergency If symptoms severe (e.g., client stuporous or comatose), progressive lethargy, or urine contains large amounts of both sugar and acetone

Cross Reference Abdominal Pain; Coma; Diabetes Mellitus; Diabetic Persons with Illness; Thirst, Excessive; Urine, Excessive Output

Special guidelines to use in treating diabetics who also have other common illnesses

Etiology

Assessment

**Treatment/
Teaching**

For diabetics with viral gastroenteritis: Maintain carbohydrate intake using 7-Up, Gatorade, orange juice, or tea with sugar. Do not use diet soft drinks during this time. Need for insulin may increase with illness (see if client is on a sliding scale or has special instructions regarding use of insulin while ill). Diabetics on a high normal dose of insulin will have a higher sliding scale. **Always** take insulin even when ill.

For diabetics with URIs: Cough syrup without sugar (e.g., ETH or ETH with codeine).

For diabetics on antibiotic therapy: Many antibiotics cause false positive urine tests on Clinitest (Keflex, Chloromycetin, and others). Use testape or Diastix for valid results.

Vitamin C doses larger than 2 Gm/day will also cause false positive urine tests.

Increased need to check for acetone in the urine when a diabetic person is ill.

Refer to MD   For evaluation of particular problem if unable to be managed at home

Emergency   If severely ill

**Cross
Reference**   Diabetic Ketoacidosis, Diabetes Mellitus, Insulin Dosage During Illness, Insulin Reaction

Increase in frequency and liquidity of stools

Etiology Intestinal infections or infestations, "nervousness," antibiotic therapy, fecal impaction, fistula, inflammatory bowel disease, carcinoma, malabsorption, pancreatic disease, biliary atresia, neurologic disease, metabolic disease, food allergy, dietary factors, overuse of laxatives, unknown

Assessment Rely on history (chronic problem vs acute onset). Check medications client is taking.

Treatment/ Teaching Clear fluids for 24 hours (e.g., Gatorade, water, 7-Up, ginger ale, broth, weak tea). When diarrhea has decreased, advance to restricted diet (nonsweetened cereals, rice, bread (not whole grain), macaroni, potatoes, yellow vegetables (squash, carrots), light-colored fruits (apples, bananas), and meats. No dairy products for 3 to 6 days. Kaopectate (3 to 6 tsp) after each loose stool prn. Watch urine output (should urinate normal amount at least every 6 to 8 hours). Monitor fever. Advance to regular diet slowly.

For diarrhea caused by antibiotics: Lactobacillus capsules or yogurt with active cultures to replace normal bowel flora.

Refer to MD For evaluation of persistent problem

Emergency Grossly bloody stool, severe abdominal pain, dehydration

Cross Reference Abdominal Pain, Blood in Stools, Colitis, Dehydration, Food Poisoning, Gastroenteritis, Rectal Bleeding, Salmonella Infection, Toxic Shock Syndrome

An acute, contagious, bacterial disease characterized by the formation of a fibrinous pseudomembrane on the mucosa, usually of the respiratory tract

Etiology   Corynebacterium diphtheriae

Assessment   Usual symptoms include fever, sore throat with tenacious gray pseudomembrane on tonsils and mucosa of throat, nasal discharge, hoarseness, malaise. The usual incubation period is from 2 to 6 days; the period of communicability is variable but rarely more than 2 to 4 weeks in untreated persons, or 1 to 2 days in persons treated with antibiotics. Diphtheria must be differentiated from streptococcal pharyngitis, infectious mononucleosis, adenovirus infection, Vincent's infection, and candidiasis.

Treatment/ Teaching   Bedrest for 3 weeks until danger of developing myocarditis has passed. Soft to liquid diet as tolerated. Saline gargles. ASA and/or codeine prn pain and fever. Prophylactic treatment for exposed persons.

Refer to MD   For diagnosis, treatment, determination of need for hospitalization

Emergency   Respiratory or cardiac distress

Cross Reference   Fever, Saline Gargle (Glossary), Sore Throat

Displacement of articular surfaces of any joint

Etiology

Assessment

**Treatment/
Teaching**

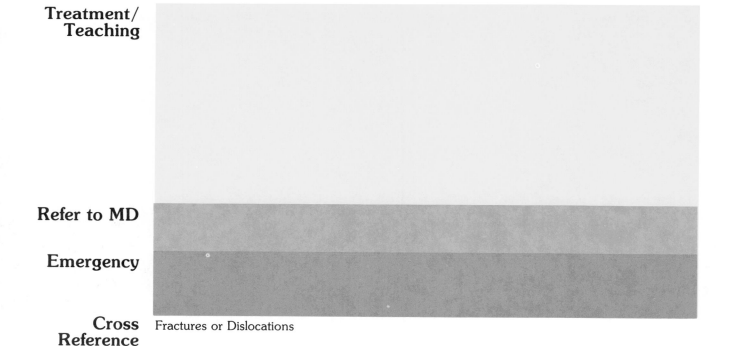

Refer to MD

Emergency

**Cross
Reference** Fractures or Dislocations

Sense of imbalance, swimming sensation; peculiar feeling in head that is not painful

Etiology   Ear infection, disturbance of equilibrium apparatus, head injury, hyperventilation, drugs, alcohol, caffeine, viral illness, cardiac problems, hypoglycemia, orthostatic hypotension, prolonged standing, motion sickness, hypertension, blood dyscrasias (e.g., anemia, leukemia), infectious diseases (e.g., measles, mumps, herpes zoster), tumors, hemorrhage, psychogenic disorders, temporal lobe seizures, multiple sclerosis

Assessment   Rely on history and ancillary symptoms. True vertigo differs from dizziness in that it refers to the sensation of objects spinning around the individual as s/he moves in relationship to surroundings, whereas dizziness is a sensation of whirling (no objects) or feeling a tendency to fall. Determine onset, if it is unremitting, positional, acute or chronic, associated with fainting, or ear symptoms.

Treatment/ Teaching   Try lying flat and quietly for 30 to 60 minutes if ancillary symptoms and history seem benign. Arise from supine position slowly, move head slowly to minimize symptoms. If no relief of symptoms after lying flat, contact MD.

Refer to MD   For evaluation and treatment prn

Emergency   Sudden onset, severe intensity, and associated with other serious ancillary symptoms

Cross Reference   Balance Problems, Ear Infection, Fainting, Head Injury, Heat Prostration, Hyperventilation, Hypoglycemia, Influenza

Seeing 2 images where 1 object actually exists

Etiology   Muscle imbalance or paralysis of 1 or more of the extraocular muscles resulting from inflammation, hemorrhage, increased intracranial pressure, trauma, infection; may be a side effect of drugs or alcohol

Assessment   Rely on history and ancillary symptoms.

Treatment/ Teaching   Expect symptoms to subside after withdrawal of drug or alcohol from client's system.

Refer to MD   For evaluation and treatment of gradual onset and nonemergency ancillary symptoms

Emergency   Sudden onset and/or history of trauma, head injury

Cross Reference

Uncontrolled salivation

Etiology CVA, blocked salivary duct, sore throat, pharyngeal abscess, foreign body aspiration, secondary effect of drugs or nausea

Assessment Rely on history and ancillary symptoms. Check for drooping of 1 side of face in evaluating possible CVA. Determine presence of any respiratory distress.

Treatment/ Teaching

Blocked salivary duct: Heat to gland and gentle massage

Foreign body aspiration: See cross reference and "Choking"

Sore Throat: See cross reference card

Refer to MD If no relief with home treatment, undiagnosed sore throat or abscess; for evaluation of CVA with mild symptoms, unaccompanied by respiratory distress; for blocked salivary duct

Emergency Severe respiratory distress, CVA with extensive symptoms

Cross Reference Choking, Epiglottitis (Peds), Sore Throat, Stroke

Sleepiness

Etiology Physical fatigue, depression, stress, head injury, medications, illness, postictal state, excessive carbohydrate intake, anemia, alcohol

Assessment Rely on history and ancillary symptoms.

Treatment/ Teaching

Physical fatigue, stress, illness: Adequate rest and relaxation.

Postictal state: Client will feel drowsy for 1 or more hours following seizure. Allow client to rest but observe for further seizure activity.

Post-head injury: Allow client to rest for 1 hour, then arouse; it is common to feel drowsy initially after head injury.

Medications: Evaluate need for medication (i.e., therapeutic value vs severity of drowsiness). If just starting a new medication, have client continue it and explain that the body frequently has to get used to a medicine, then problems will diminish.

Excess carbohydrates: Modify diet to decrease carbohydrates and increase protein intake.

Refer to MD For evaluation of persistent drowsiness and treatment of underlying problem

Emergency Prolonged drowsiness following a head injury; decreased level of consciousness; repeated seizures of increasing severity

Cross Reference Convulsions, Fatigue, Head Injury, Lethargy

Dryness, flakiness, itching secondary to decreased oil in skin

Etiology   Hereditary; use of certain soaps, cosmetics, lotions or other topical agents; excessive exposure to sun

Assessment   Differentiate from fungal infections of skin.

Treatment/ Teaching   Discontinue use of offending topical agent. Decrease number of baths; no soap or bubble baths. Moisturizers (e.g., Vaseline Intensive Care, Keri Lotion). No electric blanket.

Refer to MD   For persistent and bothersome problem not relieved with home treatment

Emergency

Cross Reference   Itching

Painful menstruation

Etiology   May be caused by release of prostaglandin in the menstrual fluid; these potent stimulators can cause pain by creating ischemia of the myometrium.

Assessment   Menstrual cramps that develop more than 5 years after menarche are usually due to organic causes. Usual symptoms include agitation, abdominal bloating, breast engorgement, pelvic heaviness, and often precede the flow. Intermittent aching to cramplike discomfort in lower abdomen usually accompanies flow. With sudden onset of pain, r/o possible abortion or ectopic pregnancy.

Treatment/ Teaching   Analgesic to manage pain (a nonsteroid, anti-inflammatory compound such as ASA or possibly ibuprofen [Motrin] to inhibit prostaglandin synthesis). Women on oral contraceptives have shown a decreased concentration of prostaglandins in their endometriums, with decreased response of the myometrium to the compounds. Heat to abdomen or back.

Refer to MD   For treatment of chronic problem and/or management of pain not relieved with home treatment

Emergency   Uterine hemorrhage (i.e., saturating a pad every 2 hours or less)

Cross Reference   Abdominal Pain, Abortion, Ectopic Pregnancy, Menorrhagia, Premenstrual Tension Syndrome

Any deviation from normal heart rhythm

Etiology   Disturbances of the automaticity of impulse-producing cells due to abnormal automatic mechanisms replacing normal rhythm; disturbances in conduction; increased awareness of normal heart action due to anxiety about presence of heart disease, or secondary to emotional disorders; other organic causes are anemia, thryotoxicosis, debility, and paroxysmal dysrhythmias.

Assessment   **Palpitations:** Brief episodes are a common complaint; without dyspnea, chest pain, fainting, weakness, or use of cardiac drugs, they are not usually dangerous. Episodes tend to last less than 10 seconds and occur in clusters over 5 to 15 minute intervals; usually occur at times of inactivity (i.e., resting after a meal or on first retiring). Two most common types of palpitations:

Sinus tachycardia—a rapid, forceful pounding that may begin gradually or suddenly but invariably slows gradually; occurs normally on exertion or during excitement.

Premature ventricular systole—causes a sensation of the heart "skipping a beat" or "stopping and turning over."

**Treatment/
Teaching**   See individual cross reference cards.

Refer to MD   For palpitations occurring in client on cardiac drugs (digitalis, quinidine, procainamide, Propanolol); to be seen same day. See in 1 to 2 days prn persistent palpitations unaccompanied by dyspnea, chest pain, fainting, weakness, or use of cardiac drugs.

Emergency   Palpitations accompanied by dyspnea, chest pain, syncope, weakness, persistent rapid palpitations, or "as though the heart were hardly beating."

**Cross
Reference**   Anemia, Angina, Atrial Fibrillation, Bradycardia, Congestive Heart Failure, Hyperventilation, Paroxysmal Atrial Tachycardia (PAT), Premature Ventricular Contractions (PVCs)

Pain in external, middle, or inner ear

Etiology Infection, pressure change, foreign body, trauma

Assessment Rely on history and ancillary symptoms. Check for presence or absence of URI, quality and nature of pain, presence or absence of any discharge from ear, plugged ears due to wax impaction, any dental/facial problems with referred otalgia (pain seeming to come from ear).

Treatment/ Teaching Analgesics (e.g., ASA or acetaminophen), saline or medicated nose drops (e.g., Afrin bid or Neo-Synephrine tid but **only** for 5 to 7 days), decongestants (e.g., Sudafed, CTM). External heat to ear. No warm oil drops in ear.

Refer to MD For fever, foreign body, or suspected trauma

Emergency Severe trauma to ear; abrupt hearing loss accompanied by pain, drainage, or dizziness

Cross Reference Earache (Peds); Ear Discharge; Ear Infection; Ear, Plugged; Ears, Ringing; Upper Respiratory Infection

Serous, sanguinous, or purulent drainage from ear canal

Etiology   Ear infection with ruptured drum, head injury, ear trauma, otitis externa ("swimmer's ear"), foreign body

Assessment   Check for history of trauma, foreign body, or head injury. Otitis externa is usually bacterial with occasional secondary fungal infection; usual symptoms are itching, pain in dry, scaling ear; may be a watery or purulent discharge and intermittent deafness. Predisposing factors are moisture in ear canal resulting from a warm, moist climate from swimming or bathing; trauma due to attempts to clean or scratch an itching ear; seborrheic and allergic dermatitis.

Treatment/ Teaching   Keep external ear clean and dry; clean with soft cloth or cotton ball, no Q-tips. No eardrops until seen by MD. Analgesics prn pain (ASA or acetaminophen). External heat to ear.

Refer to MD   Draining ear should be seen within 24 hours if infection suspected, sooner for intractable pain or foreign body

Emergency   Suspected head injury, severe ear trauma, or abrupt hearing loss accompanied by pain, drainage, or dizziness

Cross Reference   Earache; Ear Infection; Ear, Plugged; Ears, Ringing

EAR INFECTION (Otitis Externa, Otitis Media, Labyrinthitis)

Inflammation of the external, middle, or inner ear

Etiology Bacterial or fungal infection

Assessment **Otitis externa**: See "Ear Drainage."

Otitis media: Most commonly occurs in infants and children but can occur at any age; usually follows or accompanies a URI. Usual symptoms are ear pain, fever, chills, feeling of pressure or fullness in ear, decreased ability to hear; nausea and vomiting sometimes present.

Labyrinthitis: Usually follows URI; manifested by intense vertigo, marked tinnitus, a staggering gait, and nystagmus. Hearing loss often not present.

Treatment/ Teaching Analgesics prn pain (ASA or acetaminophen); may use codeine if available, either in tablet or cough syrup form if client not allergic to it. External heat to ear prn pain. No warm oil drops in ear, especially prior to exam. Elevate head. Decongestants (e.g., Sudafed, CTM). Bedrest prn dizziness.

Refer to MD For evaluation and treatment of fever and intractable pain

Emergency Abrupt hearing loss accompanied by pain, drainage, or dizziness

Cross Reference Balance Problems; Cold Symptoms; Dizziness; Earache; Ear Discharge; Ear, Plugged; Ears, Ringing; Fever; Influenza; Nausea and Vomiting

Sensation of pressure in ear and/or decreased ability to hear with or without pain.

Etiology   URI, impacted ear wax, pressure changes (e.g., airplane trips or going over mountain passes), exposure to loud noises, foreign body in ear, ear infection

Assessment   R/o recent or current URI; check for drainage from ear (serous, sanguinous, or purulent); check pain and character of pain, fever, history of trauma to ear, or chronic allergy.

**Treatment/
Teaching**

For URI or ear infection: Decongestants (Sudafed, Dimetapp). May use heat externally to ear and analgesics (ASA or acetaminophen) prn.

For impacted wax: Colace liquid in ear for 15 minutes and then wash out; one application only.

For relief of pressure changes: Pinch nostrils together and bear down as if to have BM (Valsalva's maneuver). Best method is to yawn repeatedly. Air travel not advised in presence of congestion or ear pain. If going to travel anyway, suggest decongestant and Afrin or Neo-Synephrine nose drops before flight and again before descent, if a long flight.

Refer to MD   If ear infection or foreign body suspected, if impacted wax is not relieved after single application of Colace or Debrox

Emergency   Abrupt hearing loss accompanied by pain, drainage, or dizziness

**Cross
Reference**   Earache; Ear Discharge; Ear Infection; Ears, Ringing

A buzzing, thumping, or ringing sound in ears

Etiology Toxic drug reaction to salicylates (ASA), quinine, streptomycin; foreign body in ear; Meniere's disease; infectious process in ear; cardiovascular disease; allergy; hysteria

Assessment R/o current or recent URI; check for ear pain, vomiting, medications client is taking, history of trauma to ear, history of other health problems.

Treatment/ Teaching Decongestants (e.g., Actifed, Dimetapp, Sudafed) for fluid or infection in ear. Short-term discontinuation of offending medications.

Refer to MD For evaluation and treatment

Emergency Significant hearing loss or dizziness

Cross Reference Earache; Ear Discharge; Ear Infection; Ear, Plugged

Etiology

Assessment

Treatment/
Teaching

Refer to MD

Emergency

Cross
Reference   Preeclampsia

Implantation of a fertilized ovum outside the uterine cavity

Etiology   Delayed or arrested passage of the fertilized ovum is thought to be due to defective tubal cilia, adhesions and folds of endosalpinx from previous infection and scarring, tubal diverticula, or peritubal adhesions resulting in angulation and distortion of the tube.

Assessment   Usual symptoms include skipped menstrual period or scanty flow followed by uterine bleeding, crampy pain in lower abdomen. Fainting, rectal pressure, and shoulder pain may by present. Client is rarely febrile. R/o appendicitis or other causes of acute abdomen.

Treatment/ Teaching   Treat for shock if necessary while awaiting emergency transportation.

Refer to MD   Arrange for emergency transportation to hospital

Emergency   Arrange for emergency transportation to hospital

Cross Reference   Abdominal Pain, Dysmenorrhea, Fainting, Pelvic Inflammatory Disease, Shock, Spotting

Chronic inflammation of skin, characterized by erythema, oozing, crusting, scaling, and vesicles

Etiology   May be an allergic manifestation or the result of contact with an irritant

Assessment   Distribution is characteristic with involvement of face, neck, upper trunk. The bends of elbows and knees are involved. Also appears on feet and is commonly mistaken for athlete's foot. May have family history of allergic manifestations (asthma, eczema, allergic rhinitis). Tends to recur from age 2 to early youth and beyond.

Treatment/ Teaching   Cool-water compresses to reduce itching. Keri Lotion, Nivea Cream, Lubriderm, Crisco or other solid shortenings to moisturize.

Refer to MD   For diagnosis and management of chronic symptoms

Emergency

Cross Reference   Athlete's Foot

Abnormal infiltration of tissues with fluid

Etiology   Congestive heart failure, hypertension, premenstrual fluid retention, kidney failure, pregnancy, obesity, steroid therapy, chronic illness, injury

Assessment   Evaluate for acute vs gradual onset and for evidence of cardiac and/or respiratory distress. Check client's medications to see if secondary to steroid therapy or if client is on diuretics.

Treatment/ Teaching   Elevate edematous area. Decrease salt intake. Ice pack to area if secondary to injury.

Refer to MD   For evaluation and management of underlying problem if client not in acute distress

Emergency   Cardiac or respiratory distress present

Cross Reference   Congestive Heart Failure; Preeclampsia; Pregnancy, Minor Discomforts Of

Injury resulting from the passage of electric current through the body

Etiology   Contact with electric current

Assessment   The amount and type of current, duration, area of exposure, and the pathway of current through body determine degree of damage. Direct current is much more dangerous than alternating current. Symptoms include momentary or prolonged loss of consciousness, muscle pain, fatigue, headache, nervous irritability, ventricular fibrillation, respiratory failure. Lesions are usually sharply demarcated, round or oval, painless, gray areas with inflammatory reaction. Sloughing of tissue may occur slowly over wide area after several weeks. Can cause fractures.

Treatment/ Teaching   Remove client from source of electricity. Maintain respirations and cardiac function; CPR prn until emergency aid arrives. Keep client warm.

Refer to MD   If alert and symptoms not life-threatening

Emergency   Coma, cardiac or respiratory failure

Cross Reference   Burns, Coma, Shock

A lung disease characterized by enlargement, overdistention, and destructive changes in the alveoli distal to the terminal nonrespiratory bronchioles

Etiology Smoking, heredity, unknown

Assessment Symptoms include insidious onset of exertional dyspnea (dyspnea at rest only in late stages); prolonged expiratory phase and wheezing; productive cough, often ineffective in clearing the bronchi; barrel chest, use of accessory muscles of respiration. Check for degree of symptoms and distress.

Treatment/ Teaching Use home resources, medicines, and O_2 if available. **Oxygen should run at no more than 2 liters/min** (if set higher, ask if increased rate was ordered). If client drowsy, hard to keep awake, consider CO_2 narcosis. Percussion and gravity (postural) drainage if already previously instructed.

Refer to MD For management of chronic distress prn

Emergency Severe respiratory distress unrelieved by home treatment

Cross Reference Breathing Difficulty, Cough, Cyanosis, Oxygen Information, Pulmonary Edema, Wheezing

Etiology

Assessment

Treatment/ Teaching

Refer to MD

Emergency

Cross Reference   Convulsions

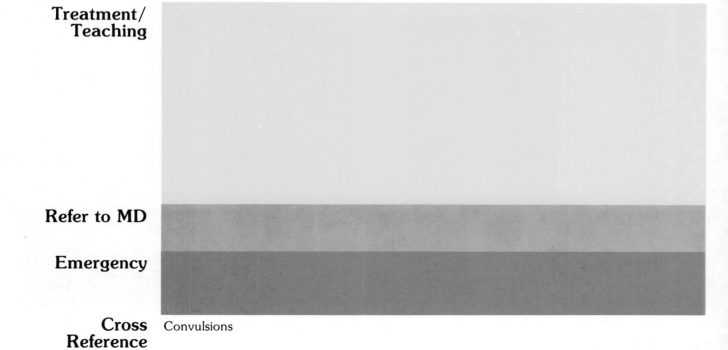

An acute inflammation of the skin and subcutaneous tissue

Etiology Beta-hemolytic streptococci

Assessment Usual symptoms include pain, malaise, fever, chills; edematous, spreading, circumscribed, hot, erythematous area with or without vesicle or bulla formation. This often occurs near a fissure at the angle of the nose.

Treatment/ Teaching Bedrest with head of bed elevated if infection occurs on face. Hot packs to affected area. ASA prn pain or fever.

Refer to MD For diagnosis and treatment with antibiotics

Emergency

Cross Reference Cellulitis, Fever, Hot Packs (Glossary), Impetigo

Arc-welding, sunburn (actinic keratitis), or ultraviolet burns of the cornea

Etiology   Excessive eye exposure to ultraviolet light

Assessment   Onset of symptoms occurs about 12 hours after exposure. Complaints consist of agonizing pain and severe photophopia.

Treatment/ Teaching   Eye rest for 48 hours (dark room or patch eyes). Cool compresses to eye prn discomfort. Analgesics, sedatives as needed. Clients recover within 24 to 48 hours without complications.

Refer to MD   For management of pain

Emergency

Cross Reference   Eye Pain

Irritation in eye caused by presence of an object

Etiology

Assessment   R/o contact lens overuse. Check corneal sensitivity to r/o herpes simplex.

Treatment/   Flush eye for 10 minutes with tepid water or saline. Soft eye patch for transportation to MD.
Teaching

Refer to MD   For removal of foreign body; evaluation and treatment of corneal abrasion

Emergency   Severe trauma, pain or visual problems, penetrating injury

Cross   Corneal Abrasion; Eye, Itching; Eye Pain; Eye Trauma
Reference

Nonpurulent, irritating, tickling sensation in the eye

Etiology   Viral infection, allergies

Assessment   R/o history of hay fever and/or allergies.

Treatment/ Teaching   Cool compresses. Antihistamines rarely useful. Visine/Murine twice a day for a few days is acceptable.

Refer to MD   If no spontaneous improvement or if secondary infection (bacterial) develops.

Emergency

Cross Reference   Conjunctivitis, Hay Fever

Mild to severe discomfort in the eye

Etiology Trauma (chemical, mechanical, or physical), infection, inflammation, sudden increase in intraocular pressure

Assessment Rely on history and ancillary symptoms. Common eye disorders that cause pain include corneal injuries, foreign bodies, infections, iritis, acute glaucoma. Check for type of pain (scratch, sharp, dull, intermittent, or continual), onset, duration, intensity, radiation, presence of photophobia, discharge, impairment of vision, redness. Neuralgia may be present as a short, sharp, one-time pain; in absence of other symptoms, this is not significant.

Treatment/ Teaching Refer to MD

Refer to MD For evaluation and treatment

Emergency Severe trauma, pain, visual problems, penetrating injury

Cross Reference Corneal Abrasion; Eye Burns; Eye Trauma; Eyes, Bloodshot; Eyes, Chemical Burns; Glaucoma; Iritis; Uveitis; Vision, Decreased

Injury to eye

Etiology   Accidents, fighting

Assessment   Rely on history and ancillary symptoms.

Treatment/   Any blow or trauma to the eye should be checked by MD.
Teaching

Refer to MD   If no sudden vision loss, bleeding, or serious injury

Emergency   Vision loss, extreme pain, hemorrhage

Cross   Eye Burns; Eye, Foreign Body; Eye Pain; Eyes, Bloodshot; Vision, Decreased
Reference

Rapid and repeated muscular contractions in eye

Etiology Irritation of nerves innervating eye muscles, fatigue (most common cause)

Assessment

Treatment/ Teaching Hot compresses to relax muscle; rest.

Refer to MD For chronic problem

Emergency

Cross Reference

Red appearance of the sclera

Etiology   Fatigue, irritants, infection, inflammation, trauma, drugs, incorrect glasses prescription, reaction to makeup or suntan lotion, allergies, tumors, increased intraocular pressure

Assessment   Rely on history and ancillary symptoms. If associated with pain, R/o iritis, glaucoma, trauma, infection.

Treatment/ Teaching   **Fatigue, mild irritation:** Cool compresses, rest.

Clear or purulent discharge: Warm compresses to eyes. Use separate towels from other family members. Avoid rubbing or scratching eyes.

Refer to MD   For evaluation of pain and/or discharge, trauma; for routine eye exam

Emergency   If associated with sudden onset of loss of vision and/or extreme pain

Cross Reference   Conjunctivitis, Eye Pain, Eye Trauma, Eye Burns, Glaucoma, Iritis

Irritation and/or damage to the eye caused by an acid or alkaline chemical

Etiology Accidental or intentional introduction of a chemical into the eye

Assessment Evaluate type of chemical. Alkali injuries are more serious and require prolonged irrigation since alkalis are not precipitated by the proteins of the eye, as are acids. Alkali burns have poorer prognosis than acid burns.

Treatment/ Teaching Immediate plain-water or saline-solution eye irrigation: 10 minutes for acid burns, 20 minutes for alkali. Check for eye pain, vision problems. Cool compresses to eyes during transport.

Refer to MD

Emergency For evaluation and immediate treatment.

Cross Reference Eye Trauma, Eye Pain

Discomfort in facial area

Etiology   Tic douloureux, herpetic infections, dental abscess or problems, sinus infections, URI, cellulitis, erysipelas

Assessment   Determine location, onset, extent, intensity, frequency, radiation, degree of pain, things that exacerbate or relieve it; presence or absence of facial paralysis, fever, other ancillary symptoms.

Treatment/ Teaching   See individual cross reference cards.

Refer to MD   If sudden onset, severe pain, facial paralysis, facial swelling and tenderness, fever, yellow or green discharge from nose

Emergency

Cross Reference   Cellulitis; Dental Problems; Erysipelas; Herpes Simplex; Shingles; Sinus Infection; Tic Douloureux

A state of temporary unconsciousness

Etiology Sensory, emotional, prolonged standing

Assessment Usual symptoms include motor weakness, epigastric distress, perspiration, restlessness, yawning, and sighing respirations. The client may appear anxious, face may be pale and cold, extremities moist. Lightheadedness, blurring of vision, and sudden loss of consciousness with decreased muscle tone may occur. R/o shock, cardiac problems, insulin shock, drug intoxication, acute alcoholism, hyperventilation, postural hypotension.

Treatment/ Teaching Place client in supine position with head lower than rest of body. Inhalation of spirits of ammonia may help revive client. Recovery should be almost immediate.

Refer to MD For recurring syncopal episodes, evaluation and treatment of cause

Emergency Cardiac symptoms, shock, or if client remains unconscious

Cross Reference Balance Problems; Dizziness; Ectopic Pregnancy; Heat Prostration; Heat Stroke; Hyperventilation; Insulin Reaction; Myocardial Infarction; Overdose, Drug; Pregnancy, Minor Discomforts Of; Shock

A feeling of tiredness, lack of energy

Etiology   Chronic illness, depression, anemia, medications, self-denial, malnutrition, depletion of energy reserves

Assessment   Symptoms include weakness, dyspnea, and weight loss. Check for evidence of depression, sense of powerlessness, history of dependence on sedatives or tranquilizers, failure to satisfy needs for rest, relaxation, recreation; earliest symptoms of congestive heart failure; heavy menstrual bleeding; history of chronic illness.

Treatment/ Teaching   Increased rest. Plan daily activities so fatigue is decreased. Well-balanced diet.

Refer to MD   For evaluation of physical complaints and/or for mental health counseling

Emergency   Severe cardiac or respiratory distress, excessive bleeding

Cross Reference   Anemia, Chest Pain, Depression, Drowsiness, Lethargy, Menorrhagia

Elevation of body temperature above normal (97 to 99°F; 36 to 37.5°C)

Etiology Infections (viral, bacterial, rickettsial, fungal, and parasitic) are the most common causes of fever. Other causes include collagen, central nervous system, malignant neoplastic, hematologic, cardiovascular, gastrointestinal, or endocrine disease; diseases due to physical (trauma, surgery) or chemical agents, disorders of fluid balance, and sometimes unknown causes.

Assessment Rely on history and ancillary symptoms.

Treatment/ Teaching **There is an association, but not yet a proved causal relationship between the use of aspirin in viral illnesses and subsequent Reye's Syndrome. Until this relationship is definitely established by the FDA, DO NOT recommend aspirin as the antipyretic agent of choice in viral illnesses, especially influenza and chickenpox (use acetaminophen) for patients 16 years of age and under.**

Antipyretic drugs (ASA or acetaminophen) every 4 hours prn temperature 101° and above, fluids, light clothing, tepid bath or shower. No alcohol sponging. Check temperature every 4 hours while awake; retake 45 to 60 minutes after antipyretic to determine effectiveness in reducing temperature. A sensation of chilling generally indicates that body temperature is increasing; perspiring usually means the fever is decreasing or "breaking." Rectal temperatures register 1° higher and axillary temperatures 1° lower than an oral temperature.

Refer to MD If a fever that has been adequately treated lasts over 48 hours (if fever is the only symptom); if other serious ancillary symptoms are present; if fever is not responding to antipyretics and home treatment

Emergency If heat stroke or thyroid crisis symptoms are present

Cross Reference Abdominal Pain; Abortion; Antipyretic Drugs; Appendicitis; Atelectasis; Balance Problems; Bladder Pain; Breast Infection; Bronchitis; Burning on Urination; Cellulitis; Chickenpox; Cold Symptoms; Convulsions; Dehydration; Delirium; Diphtheria; Ear Infection; Erysipelas; Fever (Peds); Fever, Post-op; Hallucinations; Heat Stroke; Hyperactivity; Influenza; Measles (Peds); Meningitis; Mononucleosis; Mumps; Pneumonia; Rubella; Salmonella Infection; Scarlet Fever; Shakiness; Sore Throat; Strep Throat (Peds); Swollen Glands; Thyroid Crisis; Upper Respiratory Infection

Elevated temperature occurring after surgery

Etiology   Infection; chemical agents (e.g., anesthesia); pyrogen reactions (e.g., intravenous fluids); unknown

Assessment   Rely on ancillary symptoms and history.

Treatment/ Teaching   Low grade fever (below 101°) can be expected to be present for 4 to 5 days post-op. Antipyretic every 4 hours prn temp over 101°. Light clothing. Fluids. Try to determine if surgical site is infected (presence of redness, increased tenderness, purulent drainage, streaking, swelling).

Refer to MD   For evaluation of fever, presence of infection, or other complications

Emergency

Cross Reference   Fever; Wound Infection, Post-op

Etiology

Assessment

**Treatment/
Teaching**

Refer to MD

Emergency

**Cross
Reference**   Influenza

Guidelines for management of urinary catheters in home setting

Etiology

Assessment

Urine leakage around the catheter but no urine flow into the bag may indicate a plugged catheter. If a catheter is plugged for more than 6 to 8 hours, the bladder may become distended to the point that several hours to days may be needed for bladder muscles to recover. Bladder infection is a common problem for clients with indwelling catheters. Signs of bladder infection include urine that is cloudy, foul-smelling, and contains flecks of blood or large quantities of mucus. Chills and fever may be present if there is a kidney infection.

Treatment/ Teaching

1. **Keep the catheter clean**
   a. Wash around the area where the catheter enters the body with soap and water daily, while showering or sponge bathing. An easy way to accomplish this is to sit on the toilet, use a wet washcloth to cleanse around the catheter and to wash the genital area, then pour a cup or more of warm water over the genital area to rinse.
   b. If using a leg bag, wash it each night in a 3:1 water and white vinegar solution.
   c. If using a collection bag do not clean it, only empty it from the bottom. Placing 1 aspirin a day in the bag will decrease odor.
   d. If the leg bag and collection bag are alternated, clean the inside of the collection bag with the water and white vinegar solution.
   e. Always wash hands before and after handling the catheter.
   f. When changing from leg bag to collection bag, cleanse the disconnected end of the catheter tubing with Betadine solution or soap and water.
2. **Drink plenty of fluids**
   a. Drink 1 to 2 quarts daily unless instructed otherwise.
   b. Drink fruit juices (esp. cranberry) to maintain urine acidity, help prevent infection.
   c. **If urine is dark yellow, more fluids are needed.**
3. **General instructions to prevent obstruction**
   a. Level of bag should be lower than bladder.
   b. Place tube over leg rather than under.
   c. Check for kinks and loops in tubing frequently.
   d. If urine not flowing, do not pull on catheter.
   e. Frequently "milk" the tubing or roll it between your fingers to clear an obstruction.

Refer to MD

If catheter plugged or blocked, if client is febrile, or if abdomen is distended

Emergency

Cross Reference

Urinary Tract Infection; Urine, Decreased Output or Stream

Self-limiting syndrome that develops following ingestion of food containing toxins produced by bacteria or from acute food infections; has short incubation period and a mild course

Etiology   Bacteria or toxins

Assessment   Usual symptoms include acute anorexia, nausea, vomiting, or diarrhea and cramping that is attributed to food intake, particularly if it affects groups of people and is not accompanied by fever.

Treatment/ Teaching   Nothing PO until nausea and vomiting subside, then clear fluids as tolerated. No milk if diarrhea present. Diarrhea diet prn. Report documented case to Health Department if source is believed to be a public facility.

Refer to MD   If symptoms do not subside within 48 hours, for intractable vomiting or diarrhea, if stool or food sample needed for bacteriologic exam

Emergency   Dehydration, shock, GI bleeding, suspected botulism

Cross Reference   Abdominal Pain, Blood in Stools, Blood in Vomitus, Botulism, Dehydration, Diarrhea, Gastroenteritis, Giardiasis, Nausea and Vomiting, Salmonella Infection, Shock

Guidelines for telephone management and evaluation of fractures and dislocations

Etiology   Trauma, injury

Assessment   Rely on history and ancillary symptoms.

Treatment/ Teaching   Splint area, if possible, with splint extending to joints above and below injury. Pillows work well for distal arm or leg.

Prior to transport: Ice pack for swelling, pain, and/or bleeding. Cover open wounds with sterile dressings.

Small bones: If little pain and questionable fracture and no malalignment, elevate, ice packs, check for adequacy of circulation, be seen next day.

Large bones: Client to be seen. Check for pulse in extremities. If none palpable, have client seen at closest facility.

Joints: Any trauma involving a joint needs to be seen. Check for deficit in circulation.

Toes: Tape fractured toe to next toe for support. Ice packs, elevation.

Refer to MD   For evaluation and treatment of uncomplicated fracture

Emergency   Impaired circulation, displaced fracture, dislocations, shock, hemorrhage, spinal or skull fracture

Cross Reference   Calf Pain; Cast Repair; Nose, Broken; Numbness

Freezing of skin and superficial tissues

Etiology   Exposure to extreme cold

Assessment   Flesh will be hard and white at first, then red or mottled later; may experience numbness, prickling, itching. Increased severity produces parasthesia, stiffness; thawing causes tenderness and burning pain. Skin is white or yellow and loses elasticity; edema, blisters, necrosis, and gangrene may appear.

First degree: freezing **without** blistering or peeling

Second degree: freezing **with** blistering and peeling

Third degree: freezing with necrosis of skin and possibly deeper tissue

Treatment/ Teaching   Superficial frostbite can be treated by firm steady pressure **without rubbing**. Immerse frozen portion for several minutes in water no warmer than 105°F. After normal temperature returns to the thawed area (about 1 to 1½ hours), discontinue external heat. Avoid trauma, pressure, or friction to area. Prevent infection. If skin is broken, client may need up-to-date tetanus injection.

Refer to MD   If extensive area is involved or if 2° or 3° frostbite and/or infection present

Emergency

Cross Reference

Invasion of skin by fungus

Etiology   Fungus

Assessment   Differentiate from dermatitis, psoriasis, yeast infections, eczema.

Treatment/ Teaching   Keep skin dry (moist skin favors growth of fungi). Cool climate preferred. Reduce exercise and activity to prevent excessive perspiration. Dry skin carefully after bathing or perspiring heavily. Change clothing often; wear cotton socks and underwear, sandals or open-toed shoes. Control skin secretions with talc or other drying powder. Do not overtreat with topical fungicidal agents; use ointment sparingly (many antifungal agents are strong skin irritants).

Refer to MD   If no relief with home treatment and over-the-counter antifungal agents

Emergency

Cross Reference   Athlete's Foot, Jock Itch, Ringworm

GALL BLADDER COLIC (Acute Cholecystitis)

Pain caused by inflammation of gall bladder

Etiology
Usually due to gallstones; stone becomes impacted in cystic duct and inflammation develops behind the obstruction

Assessment
Often precipitated by large or fatty meal. Characterized by sudden, severe RUQ pain (often radiating to midback or scapular area); often accompanied by nausea, vomiting, and fever. Can be confused with perforated peptic ulcer, acute pancreatitis, appendicitis in high-lying appendix, hepatitis, liver abscess, or pneumonia with pleurisy on right side.

Treatment/ Teaching
If stones previously diagnosed, clear liquids only during painful episodes; avoid fatty and/or fried foods; prescribed analgesics prn.

Refer to MD
For evaluation and management of pain, for evaluation of a new problem

Emergency

Cross Reference
Abdominal Pain, Chest Pain, Nausea and Vomiting

Guidelines for assessing need for gamma globulin therapy

Etiology

Assessment

Treatment/ Teaching

Given to persons who have been exposed to infectious hepatitis or are in daily close physical contact with the ill person (usually means only close family members). Casual social contacts or coworkers are usually not immunized unless eating facilities and bathroom facilities have been repeatedly shared with the ill person. Gamma globulin is also given to pregnant women in the first trimester of pregnancy who have a low rubella titre and have been exposed to rubella. Dosage of gamma globulin is based on weight (1 cc per 100 lb or part thereof; maximum 2 cc). Same dose schedule for adults and children. Gamma globulin can be obtained from local Health Department.

Refer to MD

If injection needed

Emergency

Cross Reference

Hepatitis, Rubella

Gas in stomach or intestines

Etiology Air swallowed during eating and drinking, gaseous foods, action of colonic bacteria, functional and organic disease of digestive system

Assessment R/o cardiac symptoms.

Treatment/ Teaching Flat 7-Up. Peppermint tea or oil of peppermint (1 drop) in tea. Knee-chest position or mild exercise (walking). Heat to abdomen. Mylicon 80, Mylanta II, or other antacid with simethicone. Avoid foods causing flatulence (beans, aromatic vegetables, carbonated beverages, milk, and milk products.) Avoid eating and drinking too rapidly and too much. Avoid laxatives and chewing gum.

Refer to MD If problem not controlled with home treatment

Emergency

Cross Reference Abdominal Pain, Belching, Bloating, Chest Pain, Heartburn, Indigestion

Acute inflammation of lining of stomach and intestine

Etiology Excessive alcohol, virus, allergy to food and drink, food poisoning, drastic cathartics, salicylates, heavy metals, infectious diseases, uremic states, extensive burns

Assessment Rely on history and ancillary symptoms. R/o appendicitis. Onset is sudden with malaise, anorexia, nausea, vomiting, abdominal cramping, diarrhea, and prostration.

Treatment/ Teaching Bedrest with convenient access to bathroom. See individual cross reference cards.

Refer to MD If no reduction in symptoms in 48 hrs; for intractable vomiting, pain; intractable diarrhea with or without GI bleeding, dehydration (mild to moderate)

Emergency Severe dehydration, extensive burns, uremia

Cross Reference Abdominal Pain, Blood in Stools, Blood in Vomitus, Diarrhea, Dehydration, Food Poisoning, Giardiasis, Nausea and Vomiting, Salmonella Infection

A form of gastroenteritis

Etiology

Giardia lamblia, a pear-shaped protozoan parasite that multiplies in the small intestine. This parasite is found most commonly in well, spring, and creek water, especially in areas endemic to beavers, who are hosts to the parasite.

Assessment

Common symptoms are nausea, flatulence, epigastric pain, abdominal cramps, distention, watery diarrhea, weight loss. History of recent hiking, skiing, or camping trip is common. R/o viral gastroenteritis, campylobacter, salmonella, staph enteritis, inflammatory bowel disease, functional or irritable bowel.

Treatment/ Teaching

Metronidazole (Flagyl) 250mg tid x 10 days after diagnosis (stool specimen for ova and parasites). Diarrhea diet (clear fluids, no milk; rice, bananas, some simple starches, bread, potatoes).

Refer to MD

For diagnosis and treatment

Emergency

Cross Reference

Abdominal Pain, Colitis, Dehydration, Diarrhea, Food Poisoning, Gastroenteritis, Salmonella Infection

A disease characterized by increased intraocular pressure and impaired vision, ranging from slight abnormalities to absolute blindness

Etiology   Unknown; predisposing factors include vasomotor and emotional instability, farsightedness, heredity, drugs

Assessment   Usually appears in persons over 40; symptoms include required, frequent change of lenses; mild headaches; vague visual disturbances; halos around electric lights; impaired adaptation to dark; eye pain. Acute attack characterized by rapid loss of sight and sudden onset of severe throbbing pain in the eye that radiates over the sensory distribution of the 5th nerve. Nausea and vomiting are frequent.

Treatment/ Teaching   Use of miotics per Rx from MD. Teach client to avoid fatigue, emotional upsets, use of tobacco, and drinking large quantities of fluids. All people over 30 should have a glaucoma pressure test approximately every 2 years.

Refer to MD   For management of chronic problem

Emergency   Sudden vision loss that may be accompanied by eye pain, headache, nausea and vomiting

Cross Reference   Eye Pain; Eyes, Bloodshot; Iritis; Vision, Decreased

An infectious venereal disease

Etiology Neisseria gonorrhoeae

Assessment **Men:** Initially, burning on urination and a serous or milky penile discharge. 1 to 3 days later, the urethral pain is more pronounced and the discharge becomes yellow, creamy, and profuse, sometimes blood-tinged.

Women: Most commonly asymptomatic. May complain of dysuria, frequency, and urgency with a purulent urethral discharge. May be only slight increase in vaginal discharge.

Treatment/ Teaching Needs treatment with antibiotics if sexual intercourse occurred with infected person or if showing symptoms. Use condom to reduce risk of infection.

Refer to MD For diagnosis and treatment; treatment also available at local Health Department

Emergency

Cross Reference Penile Discharge

Recurrent, acute arthritis of peripheral joints

Etiology Inherited metabolic disease, usually due to overproduction or underexcretion of uric acid; results from deposition of monosodium urate in and about joints and tendons

Assessment Sudden onset, frequently nocturnal; the metatarsophalangeal joint of the great toe is the most susceptible joint although those of feet, ankles, and knees are commonly affected. Pain becomes intense as involved joints become swollen, exquisitely tender with overlying skin tense, warm, and dusky red. Fever, headache, malaise, anorexia, and tachycardia are common. Client may be asymptomatic for months or years after the initial attack. May also become chronic with progressive functional loss and disability. Acute gout may be confused with cellulitis.

Treatment/ Teaching Bedrest during acute attack and for 24 hours afterward. Increased fluids to aid urate excretion. Elevate affected part and use hot or cold compresses to ease discomfort. Analgesics (frequently codeine or meperidine) prn until specific drug becomes effective. Avoid specific foods or alcoholic beverages that precipitate attacks.

Refer to MD For evaluation and treatment

Emergency

Cross Reference Cellulitis

Polyneuritis

Etiology Unknown

Assessment Polyneuritis often develops 1 to 2 weeks after a mild URI or gastroenteritis; may occur in clients recently immunized against infections such as swine influenza. Symptoms include symmetrical ascending motor weakness and distal sensory impairment, facial paralysis, difficulty with speech and swallowing. Weakness of trunk and extremity muscles may be severe. Muscle tenderness and nerve sensitivity to pressure may occur. Symptoms may progress over a week to several weeks with variable prognosis. Death may result from respiratory failure or secondary infection within a few weeks of onset. Early lower-extremity weakness extends within a few days to upper extremities and face.

Treatment/ Teaching Needs to be seen

Refer to MD If symptoms initially mild

Emergency Respiratory distress or paralysis

Cross Reference Muscle Weakness, Paralysis

False perceptions occurring without any sensory stimulus

Etiology   Drugs, alcohol, fever, narcolepsy, psychotic disorders

Assessment   Determine presence or absence of fever, use of drugs, history of psychotic disorders. Most common hallucinations are auditory or visual. In schizophrenia, the auditory hallucinations often are voices that ridicule or threaten the client in some way. Determine if client has psychotropic medications prescribed and if client has been taking them as ordered.

Treatment/ Teaching   See individual cross reference cards.

Refer to MD   For fever unresponsive to home treatment; refer to psychiatrist prn

Emergency   If hysterical or unmanageable, threatening bodily harm to self or others

Cross Reference   Confusion, Delirium, Fever, Psychosis, Suicide

Narrow strip of skin, partially detached from nail fold

Etiology Trauma, chronic irritation

Assessment

Treatment/ Teaching Trim carefully with nail scissors. Keep area clean and protected with bandaid prn.

Refer to MD If area becomes infected

Emergency

Cross Reference Nail, Infected Nailbed

Syndrome occurring after ingestion of excessive amounts of alcohol

Etiology   Excessive alcohol intake (contributed to, in part, by impurities in alcohol products e.g., histamine)

Assessment   The typical hangover headache has a throbbing quality characteristic of a vascular headache. Other symptoms include malaise, nausea, and vomiting.

Treatment/ Teaching   Bedrest. Fluids, especially fruit juices; fructose in sufficient quantity increases the rate of alcohol metabolism. When fructose is ingested with alcohol, headache is less likely to follow; when ingested during headache, its resolution is quickened. ASA or acetaminophen prn.

Refer to MD

Emergency

Cross Reference

Allergic rhinitis with catarrh of conjunctiva, nose, and throat

Etiology Exposure to pollens or other allergens

Assessment Watery nasal discharge, sneezing, itching eyes and nose. History of allergy helps distinguish allergic rhinitis from common URIs. Pollen level is highest on clear, dry days, especially in evening.

Treatment/ Teaching Antihistamines (e.g., Chlortrimeton) give relief in 60% to 80% of clients; use routinely and pre-exposure. Cool compresses for ocular itching and swelling. Maintain allergen-free atmosphere (room air filters, remove lint-producing carpets, bedspreads, etc.). Use synthetic blankets as needed if wool is allergen. Avoid feather pillows. Household pets must be considered possible source of allergens.

Refer to MD For symptoms not controlled by antihistamines and/or for desensitization or hyposensitization

Emergency

Cross Reference Allergies; Eye, Itching; Nasal Congestion

Pain in the head

Etiology   Common manifestation of acute systemic infections; stress; emotional disorders; intracranial tumors, hemorrhage, infections; head injuries; severe hypertension; cerebral hypoxia; acute or chronic diseases of the eye, nose, throat, and ear; vascular changes (migraines)

Assessment   Check for evidence of meningeal irritation (vomiting, fever, deteriorated mental state), facial pain or tenderness and/or swelling. Determine if pain is similar to head pain experienced in past, its duration and quality (i.e., persistent or episodic), history of head trauma, any neurologic irregularities. Determine the onset of pain, presence of ancillary symptoms (e.g., rhinitis, sinus congestion, ear pain, flu symptoms), presence of chronic illness (e.g., hypertension, allergies). Determine if pain is possible side effect of medications, secondary to ingestion of alcohol or tyramine (in chocolates), or due to withdrawal from coffee, cigarettes, or carbohydrates.

Migraine is characterized by paroxysmal attacks of headache often preceded by psychologic or visual disturbances and often followed by drowsiness.

Subarachnoid hemorrhage: Sudden onset, severe headache usually classified by client as "worst headache I've ever had." Unremitting in character, often accompanied by stiff neck and increasing neurologic symptoms, varying from disorientation to lethargy to coma.

Treatment/ Teaching   Analgesic (ASA or acetaminophen) every 4 hours prn pain. Lie down in dark, quiet room. Heat to posterior cervical area, cold compress to head.

Refer to MD   If no relief with over-the-counter analgesics and home treatment; for signs of head injury or if associated with acute infection or chronic problems requiring further evaluation

Emergency   Intractable pain with or without vomiting and fever; marked mental or neurologic deterioration; unequal pupils

Cross Reference   Hangover, Head Injury, Heat Prostration, Heat Stroke, Hypertension, Influenza, Meningitis, Migraine Headache, Sinus Congestion

Traumatic damage to the skull and its contents

Etiology A fall or blow to the head with an object

Assessment History of fall or blow to the head makes cause of unconsciousness evident; if history of trauma is absent, differentiate head injury from other causes of unconsciousness (e.g., diabetes, hepatic or alcoholic coma, CVA, or epilepsy where trauma to head may have occurred during seizure).

Treatment/ Teaching Evaluation of any head injury should include 24-hour observation of the client for the following symptoms, with instruction for client to be brought in if any occur:

1. Decreased level of consciousness; excessively difficult to arouse or markedly restless. Drowsiness is common initially after head injury. Let client sleep for an hour, then arouse. Awaken every 2 to 3 hours during night to monitor responsiveness.

2. Vomiting occurring more than once or projectile vomiting

3. Unequal and/or unresponsive pupils. Have observer check client's pupils with flashlight for reactivity and equality.

4. Headache unrelieved by ASA or acetaminophen

5. Serous or sanguinous drainage from nose, mouth, or ears

6. Slurred speech, lack of coordination and balance

7. Unexplained fever

8. Convulsions

9. Inability to move arms and legs on either side

For mild head injury without loss of consciousness, client should have quiet activity or bedrest for 24 hours. May use icepack if "goose egg" develops.

Refer to MD If client initially unconscious, if any of the above symptoms develop, or if suturing needed

Emergency Coma, hemorrhage, convulsions, severe trauma

Cross Reference Balance Problems, Coma, Confusion, Convulsions, Dizziness, Drowsiness, Ice Pack (Glossary), Irritability, Nausea and Vomiting

Eructation of gastric acid contents into mouth accompanied by a burning sensation

Etiology   Hiatus hernia, indigestion, pregnancy, cardiac problem

Assessment   R/o cardiac symptoms.

Treatment/ Teaching   Take antacids 1 hour and 3 hours after eating and at bedtime in 1 to 2 tbsp doses (liquid antacids best). Antacids containing magnesium (e.g., Maalox and Mylanta) may cause loose bowels. Antacids containing aluminum (e.g., Gelusil and WinGel) may constipate. Riopan may be used by those on low sodium diet. Tums are very effective. For heartburn during pregnancy, recommend calcium carbonate antacids (Tums). Discontinue spices, coffee, smoking, tea, alcohol, carbonated drinks, and chocolate. Avoid milk if gastric juices seem to be increased. Eat small, dry meals. Elevate head of bed, avoid eating and drinking 2 to 3 hours before bedtime. Maintain erect posture after eating. Avoid tight clothing (e.g., girdles and belts).

Refer to MD   For evaluation and treatment of continuing problem unrelieved by home treatment

Emergency   Cardiac symptoms

Cross Reference   Belching; Gas; Hiatus Hernia; Indigestion; Myocardial Infarction; Pregnancy, Minor Discomforts Of

Etiology

Assessment

**Treatment/
Teaching**

Refer to MD

Emergency

**Cross
Reference** Angina, Atrial Fibrillation, Bradycardia, Chest Pain, Congestive Heart Failure, Dysrhythmias, Myocardial Infarction, Paroxysmal Atrial Tachycardia, Premature Ventricular Contractions

Syndrome characterized by prostration and varying degrees of circulatory collapse

Etiology   Exposure to excessive heat resulting in inadequacy or collapse of the peripheral circulation secondary to dehydration and salt depletion

Assessment   Symptoms are weakness, dizziness, stupor, and headache, with or without muscle cramps. The skin is cool and pale, vision is dim or blurred. Mental confusion and muscular incoordination may occur. All symptoms are usually transient and prognosis excellent.

Treatment/ Teaching   Place client in cool place in reclining position; elevate feet. Give water if alert and able to swallow.

Prevention: Increase salt and fluid intake in hot weather. Decrease activity at peak of heat.

Refer to MD   If client not responding rapidly to treatment

Emergency   Acute circulatory failure

Cross Reference   Dehydration, Dizziness, Headache, Heat Stroke

Acute dermatitis occurring most commonly on upper extremities, trunk, and intertriginous areas

Etiology Hot, moist environment is most common cause

Assessment Burning, itching, superficial, aggregated, small vesicles or papules on covered areas of skin; distinguish from similar skin manifestations occurring from a drug reaction.

Treatment/ Teaching Reduce clothing; cool bath; put cornstarch in bath water and on rash. Avoid overbathing and use of strong irritating soaps. Control temperature, ventilation, and humidity.

Refer to MD For secondary infection or severe reaction

Emergency If associated with heat prostration

Cross Reference Cornstarch Bath (Glossary), Rash

Syndrome characterized by sudden loss of consciousness and by failure of the body's heat-regulating mechanisms

Etiology Usually follows excessive heat exposure or strenuous physical activity under hot atmospheric conditions, although it may develop in elderly, infirm, or otherwise susceptible individuals in absence of unusual heat exposure

Assessment There may be premonitory headache, dizziness, nausea, confusion, convulsions, and visual disturbances that progress to coma. The skin is hot, flushed, and usually dry; pulse is strong and rapid. Rectal temperature may be as high as 109°F (42.6°C) (brain protein denatures at 106°F [41°C]).

Treatment/ Teaching Place client in cool, shady place and remove all clothing. Sponge with tepid water while awaiting emergency transportation.

Refer to MD Arrange emergency transportation to hospital

Emergency Arrange emergency transportation to hospital

Cross Reference Convulsions, Fever, Headache, Heat Prostration

A soft tissue swelling filled with blood

Etiology   Trauma

Assessment   Rely on history and ancillary symptoms.

Treatment/ Teaching   Area will remain painful, swollen, and discolored for some time. Apply ice pack or cold compress (20 minutes at a time, 4 times a day) for 24 to 72 hours depending on severity of hematoma; then moist heat for 20 minutes, 4 times a day, if it does not produce new swelling. Symptoms should resolve within 3 to 4 weeks following injury.

Refer to MD   As needed for signs of infection or for evaluation

Emergency   Dramatically increased swelling

Cross Reference   Bruise, Ice Pack (Glossary)

Varicosity of veins around anus

Etiology Straining at stool, constipation, prolonged sitting, pregnancy, and infection are contributing factors

Assessment Usual complaints include rectal pain or itching, protrusion of veins, rectal bleeding, mucoid rectal discharge. Hemorrhoidal bleeding usually produces streaks of blood on stool surface but bleeding can be more profuse.

Treatment/ Teaching Tucks, Preparation H, sitz baths, bedrest, hemorrhoidal suppositories, manual reduction of hemorrhoid prn. Avoid prolonged sitting, standing, lifting, straining. Keep stools soft with high roughage diet, increased fluid intake, and stool softener (per order of MD). To treat or prevent itching, wash anal area with clear, warm water and pat dry after each BM.

Refer to MD For pain unrelieved by home treatment, increased rectal bleeding with stools or rectal bleeding in absence of stool, incontinence, signs of infection

Emergency

Cross Reference Blood in Stools; Pregnancy, Minor Discomforts Of; Rectal Bleeding

Inflammation of the liver

Etiology Viral infection occurring sporadically or in epidemics. There are 3 types of hepatitis: A, B, and non-A/non-B (rare). A is transmitted from person to person by the fecal-oral route. Hepatitis B is usually transmitted by inoculation of infected blood or blood products, but can be transmitted in any body fluid (e.g., semen).

Assessment Usual symptoms include anorexia, nausea, vomiting, malaise, symptoms of upper respiratory infection or "flu-like" syndrome, RUQ tenderness or pain, fever, clay-colored stools, dark urine, jaundice, loss of taste for cigarettes in a smoker. R/o URI, influenza. Severity of disease is directly correlated with the client's age; children may have subclinical cases.

Treatment/ Teaching Bedrest during the initial phase. Give palatable meals and increase fluid intake. No alcohol for 6 months. Wash hands well after bowel movement and after contact with contaminated utensils, bedding, or clothing. Gamma globulin should be given within 2 to 3 weeks to persons in a close living situation with the client.

Refer to MD For diagnosis and management to assess the need for hospitalization, especially of those dehydrated due to severe anorexia and vomiting

Emergency

Cross Reference Abdominal Pain; Gamma Globulin Information; Jaundice; Stools, Light-Colored; Nausea and Vomiting; Urine, Dark-Colored

Abnormal protrusion of organ or part of an organ through an aperture in the surrounding structures

Etiology   Straining, heavy lifting, tissue weakness

Assessment   In the case of hiatus hernia, r/o cardiac symptoms. Strangulated inguinal hernia is characterized by severe pain at the hernia site with a firm, tender mass that cannot be reduced; frequently accompanied by nausea and/or vomiting.

Treatment/ Teaching   **Umbilical or inguinal hernia:** Avoid heavy lifting, straining. Try to reduce by lying down and gently pushing hernia in.

Hiatus hernia: See cross reference card

Refer to MD   If unable to reduce hernia or if severe pain present

Emergency

Cross Reference   Hiatus Hernia

Vesicular lesions on genitals, sometimes on mouth

Etiology Herpes virus types I and II, transmitted sexually

Assessment Typical lesions are multiple, shallow ulcerations, vesicles, and erythematous papules. Females may complain of fever, malaise, anorexia, local genital pain and/or itching, leukorrhea, dysuria, and sometimes vaginal bleeding. Males may complain of pruritus until lesions ulcerate or secondary infection occurs, then lesions are painful. R/o syphilis.

Treatment/ Teaching
Males: Keep genital area clean. Nupercainal ointment prn discomfort until seen by MD. Abstain from sexual intercourse while lesions are present. Condoms offer some protection.

Females: Sitz bath, cold compresses prn discomfort. Nupercainal ointment prn discomfort until seen by MD. ASA or codeine prn pain (check for allergy to codeine). Abstain from sexual intercourse while lesions are present.

Refer to MD For diagnosis and treatment, for secondary infection, for pronounced dysuria

Emergency

Cross Reference Penile Lesion, Vaginal Itching, Voiding Difficulty

Vesicular eruption, particularly circumorally

Etiology Herpes simplex virus

Assessment Clinical outbreaks, which may be recurrent in the same location for years, are provoked by fever, sunburn, indigestion, fatigue, windburn, menstruation, or nervous tension. Symptoms include small, grouped vesicles in an erythmatous base, especially around oral and genital areas. Regional lymph nodes may be swollen and tender. R/o herpes zoster (shingles), impetigo.

Treatment/ Teaching Cold compresses or ice packs to lesions for comfort.

In mouth: Popsicles, ice chips, fluids. Benadryl/Maalox mix as mouthwash/gargle. Gly-Oxide directly to lesions.

Outside mouth: Camphophenique, Blistex, on lesions; avoid touching since virus can be spread. Wash hands after contact with lesion.

Refer to MD For multiple lesions, management of discomfort, or symptoms of eye infection

Emergency

Cross Reference Benadryl-Maalox (Glossary); Cold Sore; Herpes, Genital; Sore Throat; Shingles

Protrusion of stomach above the diaphragm through esophageal opening

Etiology   Unknown; may be congenital or secondary to trauma

Assessment   Midsternal, burning sensation occurring after meals ("feels like heartburn"); may be relieved by antacids. May occur when bending or lying down, often awakens client at night. R/o cardiac symptoms.

Treatment/ Teaching   When picking something off the floor, bend at the knees, not the hips; avoid bending over, lifting, straining at stool. Elevate head of bed on blocks. Small frequent meals. Antacids (e.g., Gaviscon, Mylanta) after meals and between meals. Avoid tight clothing around the midsection, low chairs that cause slumping, smoking; do not eat food less than 3 hours before bedtime.

Refer to MD   For evaluation and management if not relieved by home treatment

Emergency   Severe abdominal distress or pain, internal bleeding

Cross Reference   Abdominal Pain, Belching, Chest Pain

Involuntary spasmodic contraction of the diaphragm followed by sudden closure of glottis producing a characteristic sound

Etiology Result of irritation of afferent or efferent nerves or of medullary centers controlling muscles of respiration, particularly the diaphragm

Assessment Check for cardiac symptoms. R/o CNS disorders, cardiorespiratory disorders, infectious diseases. May be the only symptom of peptic esophagitis. Can be a subtle symptom of pulmonary embolus in predisposed client.

Treatment/ Teaching Rebreathe into paper bag. Plug nose and ears and drink glass of water. Stroke back of tongue. Swallow spoonful of dry sugar. Take antacids.

Refer to MD If no relief with home treatment or if recurrent and persistent

Emergency

Cross Reference

Discomfort or pain initiating from or referred to the hip area

Etiology Bursitis, arthritis, fracture or trauma, renal calculi, pinched nerve or low back pain, infection, tendonitis

Assessment Bursitis is usually a pain felt laterally whereas arthritis pain is usually felt in the groin. Check for fever, history of trauma or fall, frequency and nature of pain, onset, history of similar pain, things that exacerbate or relieve it, radiation, degree of activity limitation due to pain. Check for urinary symptoms (dysuria, urgency, hesitancy, frequency, hematuria).

Treatment/ Teaching Rest; heat or ice pack; ASA or acetaminophen prn discomfort.

Refer to MD For persistent pain unrelieved by home treatment; evaluation of trauma or fall; urinary symptoms

Emergency Severe pain and/or inability to move or bear weight on leg; displaced fracture

Cross Reference Arthritis, Bursitis, Kidney Stones

An allergic skin eruption characterized by multiple, circumscribed, smooth, raised, pinkish, itchy wheals developing very suddenly, usually lasting a few days, and leaving no visible trace after resolution

Etiology Drug allergy, insect stings or bites, desensitization injections (allergy shots), allergy to certain foods (especially eggs, shellfish, nuts, fruits)

Assessment Exposure to or ingestion of known allergen versus contact dermatitis. Determine extent of reaction. In searching for etiology, it is helpful to record all intake for previous 12 to 24 hours in addition to drug, insect, plant, inhalant exposure. Check for respiratory difficulty, wheezing.

Treatment/ Teaching Oral antihistamines (e.g., CTM, Benadryl) every 4 to 6 hours until symptoms are gone. Cool baths and showers, cool baking soda baths, Calamine lotion. Stay out of sun. If drug related, discontinue drug and have client report to MD. Eliminate cause if possible.

Refer to MD If no response to home treatment; for evaluation of cause

Emergency Anaphylactic reaction (i.e., parasthesia, choking, cyanosis, wheezing, facial edema, shock, loss of consciousness, convulsions, fever, cough, incontinence)

Cross Reference Allergic Reaction, Severe; Allergies; Allergy Shot Reaction; Ampicillin/Amoxicillin Rash (Peds); Anaphylaxis; Dermatitis, Contact

Change in the quality or quantity of the voice due to interference with vibration, approximation, or tension of the vocal cords

Etiology Infectious process, neurologic disorder, tumor, trauma, allergy, metabolic and endocrine disorders

Assessment Rely on history and ancillary symptoms.

Treatment/ Teaching Rest voice. Warm or cool saline gargles, whichever feels best. Vaporizer. Clear fluids. Discontinue smoking. Steam breathing (turn hot water on in sink, place head down with towel over head and breathe the steam).

Refer to MD For evaluation and treatment if persists more than 48 hours

Emergency Severe respiratory distress

Cross Reference Anaphylaxis, Cold Symptoms, Saline Gargle (Glossary), Sore Throat

Excessive activity

Etiology	Drugs, withdrawal from alcohol or coffee, ingestion of excess sugar or red dye, thyroid problems, fever, emotional problems, behavior disorders
Assessment	Rely on history and ancillary symptoms. Investigate client's medications.
Treatment/ Teaching	Antipyretics (e.g. ASA, acetaminophen), tepid bath, light clothing if fever is cause. Discontinue any medication that may be suspect.
Refer to MD	For chronic problem or if alcohol- or drug-related
Emergency	Symptoms sudden and severe
Cross Reference	Anxiety, Fever

HYPERTENSION (High Blood Pressure)

Abnormally high systolic and diastolic levels (chiefly the latter, especially if over 90 mm Hg)

Etiology

In 90% of cases, no cause can be established ("essential hypertension"). It affects 10% to 15% of white adults and 20% to 30% black adults in US. Onset between 25 to 55 years of age. Elevations are transient in early course of disease, but eventually become permanent. Heredity and ingestion of large amounts of salt are implicated as predisposing factors.

Assessment

Primary hypertension may be present for years in asymptomatic form. Clients may complain of fatigue, nervousness, dizziness, palpitations, insomnia, weakness, and headache. Hypertension considered present if diastolic pressure consistently exceeds 100 mm Hg in a person more than 60 years old or 90 mm Hg in person less than 50 years. Hormones and birth control pills can induce hypertension; check if client on these meds.

Treatment/ Teaching

Sodium-restricted diet; discontinue caffeine, nicotine, alcohol, licorice, cold tablets; no antihistamines. If recent cataract surgery and client on eye drops, lower sodium intake and increase fluids prn. Hypertensive clients are more prone to CVA, MI, kidney stones and other kidney disease. Consider client's anxiety level. Suggest bananas and orange juice for potassium deficiency due to antihypertensive meds (i.e., diuretics).

Refer to MD

For evaluation, if diastolic over 100 mm Hg, for potassium deficiency due to antihypertensive meds, if hypertension seems drug-related, or if current prescription for tranquilizers and antihypertensives are not controlling pressure

Emergency

Cardiac complications secondary to hypertension

Cross Reference

Condition due to excessive production of thyroid gland hormone

Etiology Unknown; familial tendency often present

Assessment One of most common endocrine disorders; highest incidence in women ages 20 to 40. Symptoms include restlessness, nervousness, irritability, easy fatigability (especially toward end of day), unexplained weight loss in spite of ravenous appetite, excessive sweating, heat intolerance, quick, uncoordinated movements, fine tremor, velvety skin, and silky hair. When associated with diffuse goiter and ocular irregularities, it is called Graves' disease.

Treatment/ Teaching

Refer to MD For evaluation and treatment

Emergency Signs of thyroid crisis

Cross Reference Hypothyroidism, Shakiness, Swollen Glands, Thyroid Crisis or Storm, Thyroid Replacement Therapy

Rapid deep breathing, panting, but not dyspneic

Etiology Pain, anxiety, emotional problems

Assessment Client usually under stress or beset with emotional problems; may complain of dizziness, numbness, tingling in face and arms, feeling of suffocation or tightness in chest; may/may not be accompanied by awareness of respiratory distress. Symptoms may last up to 30 minutes and occur several times a day.

Treatment/ Teaching Rebreathe into paper bag for 5 to 10 minutes. Pattern of breathing is unimportant. If symptoms recur or are incompletely controlled after 5 to 10 minutes, breathe room air for 5 minutes, then repeat. If the use of a paper bag is precluded for some reason, have client breathe shallowly 12 times/minute or 1 breath every 5 seconds (time by a second hand on a timepiece).

Refer to MD For evaluation of underlying problem or if no relief with home treatment

Emergency

Cross Reference Anxiety, Balance Problems, Dizziness, Fainting, Numbness

Abnormally decreased blood sugar

Etiology   Secondary manifestation of nervous system imbalance; vagal overactivity causing increased gastric emptying and early hyperinsulinism in response to a meal, specific nutrients or drugs, including alcohol; fasting

Assessment   Symptoms usually occur several hours after eating and include sweating, flushing or pallor, numbness, chilliness, hunger, trembling, headache, dizziness, weakness, palpitations; may have elevated pulse rate, nausea, apprehensiveness, and syncope. The severe hypoglycemic may act drunk or exhibit bizarre behavior.

Treatment/ Teaching   Reduce proportion of carbohydrates in diet. Avoid refined sugar. Increase the frequency and reduce the size of meals (5 or 6 small feedings per day). High protein foods recommended.

Refer to MD   For evaluation and further treatment if necessary

Emergency   Convulsion and/or coma

Cross Reference   Balance Problems, Coma, Convulsions, Dizziness, Insulin Reaction

HYPOTHYROIDISM

Syndrome caused by decreased thyroid hormone output

Etiology   Thyroidectomy, radiation therapy to neck, atrophy of gland from unknown causes

Assessment   Most common symptoms are weakness, fatigue, cold intolerance, lethargy, dryness of skin, constipation, and menorrhagia. Nails may be thin and brittle, hair may be thinning out but coarse in texture, skin may have pallor. Mild hypothyroidism must be considered in all states of neurasthenia, menstrual disorders without grossly demonstrable pelvic disease, unexplained weight gain, and anemia.

Treatment/ Teaching   Determine if client on thyroid replacement therapy

Refer to MD   For evaluation and treatment

Emergency

Cross Reference   Hyperthyroidism, Shakiness, Thyroid Crisis, Thyroid Replacement Therapy

Guidelines for adult immunization

Etiology

Assessment

Treatment/ Teaching

Rabies: Check with own MD or health department.

Rubella (German measles): In a pregnant woman, can cause severe defects in the unborn child. Any woman of childbearing age should be absolutely sure she is not pregnant before being given the rubella vaccine. Wait 3 months after dose of vaccine to become pregnant.

Rubeola (red measles): Highly recommended for those under 25 years of age or any adult born after 1956 who has no prior history of having rubeola. If vaccinated prior to 1968, reimmunize.

Smallpox vaccination: No longer given in US. For current requirements for overseas travel immunizations, check with local health department.

Tetanus booster: With injury, need to have had initial series (as a child) and a booster within the past 5 years. If no injury, routine immunization every 10 years. Clients with no history of tetanus immunization who have an injury (i.e., trauma or bite) need to be seen immediately. Clients with tetanus immunization history but needing a booster should be seen within 72 hours of the injury. If the client has not had the initial series, human tetanus antitoxin should be given as well as the first immunization of the series. The schedule for completion of series: 2nd dose 4 to 6 weeks after 1st dose, and 3rd dose 6 to 12 months after 2nd dose.

Refer to MD

As indicated above

Emergency

For exotic vaccines (e.g., snake bite antivenin); can be obtained through (fill in information applicable to your area):

Cross Reference

Bites, Animal and Human (Peds); Gamma Globulin Information; Immunization Information (Peds); Mumps; Tetanus Immunization (Peds)

An inflammatory, pustular, oozing, crusting skin disease often around the nose and mouth

Etiology Staphylococcus or streptococcus

Assessment Pruritic lesions consisting of macules, vesicles, pustules, and honey-colored, gummy crusts that leave denuded, red areas when removed. The face and other exposed parts most often involved. Contagious, infected material may be transmitted to skin by dirty fingernails. R/o herpes simplex, chickenpox, contact dermatitis.

Treatment/ Teaching Topical antibiotics may be used on small, new lesions. For lesions unresponsive to topical therapy or for large lesions, oral antibiotics are the treatment of choice. In clients where post-streptococcal glomerulonephritis is a consideration, oral antibiotics will probably be used initially. Gentle debridement by washing with soap and water 2 or 3 times a day. Cover hands with socks if child can't stop scratching and cut nails maximally. May prophylactically coat anterior nares of child with Bacitracin to prevent spreading to other areas from child "picking his nose."

Refer to MD For diagnosis or if infection spreading

Emergency

Cross Reference Cold Sore, Lip Lesions, Erysipelas

Inability to control evacuation of urine

Etiology Anatomic abnormality, physical stress, UTI, CVA, prostatitis, spinal cord injury, retention, overflow incontinence

Assessment Rely on history and ancillary symptoms. Determine if an acute or chronic problem.

Treatment/ Teaching Keep perineum as clean and dry as possible to prevent break-down of tissue. Use a pad inside underwear; rubber sheet or large piece of plastic under regular sheet to protect bedding. Never tie a bag around the penis; use condom-style catheter if appropriate.

Refer to MD For acute problem or management of chronic one

Emergency

Cross Reference Prostatitis, Stroke, Urinary Tract Infection

A symptom complex including nausea, heartburn, upper abdominal pain, flatulence and eructation, a sense of fullness, and a feeling of abdominal distention, occuring during or after the ingestion of food

Etiology   Eating too much or too rapidly, inadequate mastication, eating during emotional upsets or severe mental strain, swallowing large amounts of air, excessive smoking, excessive caffeine, constipation, ingestion of poorly cooked, high fat-content food and gas-forming vegetables

Assessment   R/o cardiac symptoms.

Treatment/ Teaching   Eat well-balanced diet without haste, in relaxing environment, and in moderate amounts. Refrain from smoking immediately before meals. Avoid excitement following a meal. Avoid gum chewing to decrease volume of air swallowed. Antacids.

Refer to MD   For evaluation of chronic problem unrelieved by home treatment

Emergency   Cardiac symptoms

Cross Reference   Abdominal Pain, Belching, Bloating, Gas, Heartburn, Myocardial Infarction

Highly contagious, acute infection

Etiology   Viral

Assessment   Influenza is transmitted by the respiratory route; the incubation period is from 1 to 4 days. The onset is usually abrupt with fever, chills, malaise, prostration, muscular aching, substernal soreness, headache, nasal stuffiness, occasional nausea, coryza, nonproductive cough, and sore throat. Fever lasts 1 to 7 days (usually 3 to 5). Diagnosis is difficult in the absence of a classic epidemic because it resembles many other mild febrile illnesses, but is usually accompanied by a cough.

Treatment/ Teaching   Bedrest. Clear fluids. Acetaminophen prn fever and aches (refer to Antipyretic Drugs). Light clothing if febrile. Decongestant (e.g., Sudafed, Chlotrimeton) prn nasal congestion. Expectorant (e.g., 2/G, Robitussin) prn cough.

Refer to MD   For evaluation and treatment of secondary infections or complications (e.g., sinusitis, otitis media, bronchitis, pneumonia)

Emergency

Cross Reference   Antipyretic Drugs, Aspirin and Acetaminophen (Peds), Bronchitis, Dizziness, Ear Infection, Nausea and Vomiting, Pneumonia, Sinus Infection, Upper Respiratory Infection

Outer margins of nail plates buried in the nail fold

Etiology Improperly trimmed toenail, tight shoes that do not allow good ventilation of the feet

Assessment

Treatment/ Teaching Warm, soapy soaks. Cut nail straight across, not in rounded shape. Try small cotton pledget under corner of nail plate to encourage corner of nail plate to grow free beyond nail groove. Elevate foot to prevent swelling.

Refer to MD If infection develops, if discomfort continues, if surgical intervention necessary

Emergency

Cross Reference

Sleeplessness

Etiology Situational problems such as transient stress, job pressures, marital discord; medical disorders that include pain and physical discomfort; drug-related episodes, including withdrawal from alcohol or sedatives; psychologic conditions

Assessment Rely on history and ancillary symptoms.

Treatment/ Teaching Hot shower or tub bath, herbal teas, hot drink, warm milk, exercise, reading, listening to soothing music. Instruct client how to take sedatives if already has prescription for same.

Refer to MD For evaluation and management of chronic problem

Emergency

Cross Reference Anxiety

Not for Day-to-Day Regulation

Etiology   The need for insulin usually is increased by illness.

Assessment

Treatment/ Teaching

1. At the first sign of illness, check the urine for glucose before each meal and at bedtime, using Clinitest or Ketodiastix. Record the results.

   RESULTS:

Clinitest (glucose)	Ketodiastix (glucose)	Color	Ketodiastix (Ketones)	Color
trace	$\frac{1}{10}$%	Blue	Negative	Tan
+	$\frac{1}{4}$%		small	
+ +	$\frac{1}{2}$%	↓	medium	↓
+ + +	1%		large	
+ + + +	2%	Brown		Purple

2. Continue to take usual insulin injections each day. Never omit the usual dosage of insulin even if nauseated and vomiting. THE NEED FOR INSULIN USUALLY IS INCREASED BY ILLNESS.

3. Take extra insulin if feeling ill and tests show 2% glucose or higher. Check urine before each meal and at bedtime. Each time glucose level is 2%, take extra units of regular insulin. To calculate the amount of insulin to be taken, add the number of units usually taken each day (include all mixtures), divide the total by 4, and administer this amount prn.

4. If nauseated, substitute bland or liquid foods for usual diet. To avoid ketoacidosis and possible hypoglycemia, clients who take insulin must consume at least 150 grams of carbohydrates each day. 1½ quarts of fluid containing sugar (ginger ale, cola, fruit juice) taken in small amounts over a 24-hour period will satisfy this requirement.

Refer to MD   If condition gets worse (i.e., illness lasts longer than 24 hours), vomiting continues, ketones persist in urine, for any questions

Emergency

Cross Reference   Diabetic Persons with Illness

INSULIN REACTION (Diabetic Hypoglycemia)

Decreased blood sugar level in diabetics receiving insulin

Etiology Delay or omission of a meal, increase in exercise, period of emotional stress, excess dose of insulin

Assessment May complain of headache, weakness; skin may be moist and pale. Client may drool, breathing will be normal or shallow; acetone odor on breath is rare. The onset is usually sudden.

Treatment/ Teaching If client conscious, give table sugar, orange or grape juice, or candy. Check urine for ketones. Remind client to carry some form of sugar with him at all times.

Refer to MD If problem is recurrent and frequent, or no improvement with ingestion of sugar

Emergency Coma

Cross Reference Diabetes Mellitus, Diabetic Ketoacidosis, Diabetic Persons with Illness, Fainting, Hypoglycemia

Inflammation of the iris

Etiology Trauma; possible infectious, toxic, or metabolic process in eye

Assessment Rapid onset of redness, deep eye pain, photophobia, and discomfort or pain about the entire orbit up into the frontal-temporal bones; usually unilateral. There may be edema of the upper lid, tearing, blurred vision, transient myopia; iris appears dull and swollen (brown irises become muddy; blue or gray ones look greenish). R/o glaucoma, conjunctivitis, corneal ulcer.

Treatment/ Teaching

Refer to MD For evaluation and treatment

Emergency Severe pain or visual disturbances

Cross Reference Conjunctivitis; Eyes, Bloodshot; Eye Pain; Glaucoma, Primary; Uveitis

Change in normal bowel pattern

Etiology

Assessment

**Treatment/
Teaching**

Refer to MD

Emergency

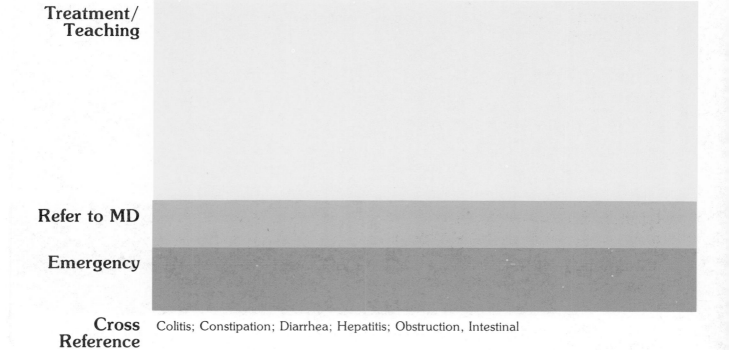

**Cross
Reference**　　Colitis; Constipation; Diarrhea; Hepatitis; Obstruction, Intestinal

Excessive reaction to slight stimulation; impatient, easily angered, exasperated, or excited

Etiology CVA, head injury, medications, illness, alcohol ingestion, emotional problems

Assessment Rely on history and ancillary symptoms.

Treatment/ Teaching Establish a calm, low-stimulus environment. Assess need for mental health counseling.

Refer to MD For evaluation of cause, if not accompanied by emergency symptoms

Emergency Sudden and dramatic change in behavior and/or if accompanied by other symptoms requiring urgent attention (e.g., violent behavior, injury, change in level of consciousness)

Cross Reference Head Injury, Stroke

A disagreeable sensation, inducing the desire to scratch

Etiology Dermatologic disorders, idiopathic, excessive dryness of skin, pressure, chafing, chemical irritants, contact and other allergies, emotional factors, viral rashes, pregnancy

Assessment Rely on history and ancillary symptoms.

Treatment/ Teaching If skin is dry, bathe and apply emollient. Tepid tub bath, baking soda in water; avoid bubble bath; blot dry (don't rub). Avoid overbathing, prolonged bath periods, exposure to drafts after bathing. Calamine lotion prn relief. Oral antihistamines prn.

Refer to MD For evaluation of persistent problem

Emergency

Cross Reference Allergies, Chickenpox, Cornstarch Bath (Glossary), Dry Skin, Hives, Lice, Nettles Contact, Oatmeal Bath (Glossary), Pinworms, Poison Oak or Ivy, Scabies, Ticks

A condition characterized by a raised bilirubin level in the blood with deposition of pigment in skin

Etiology   Common causes include hepatitis, alcoholism with cirrhosis, drug ingestion, hemolytic anemia, infectious mononucleosis

Assessment   Rely on history and ancillary symptoms; differentiate acute from chronic problem.

Treatment/ Teaching

Refer to MD   For evaluation and treatment

Emergency

Cross Reference   Hepatitis, Itching, Mononucleosis

Infection of the groin and gluteal cleft

Etiology   Fungus

Assessment   Lesion consists of erythematous macules with sharp margins, cleared centers, and active, spreading peripheries in intertriginous areas; may have vesicles at borders; itching usually more severe than with seborrheic dermatitis but less than with psoriasis of groin area. Differentiate from psoriasis, seborrheic dermatitis, or monilia. May have associated tinea infection of feet (i.e., "Athlete's Foot").

Treatment/ Teaching   Keep area clean and dry; avoid overbathing. Apply Cruex, Desinex, Tinactin, or Zeasorb powder. Wear white cotton boxer shorts.

Refer to MD   If secondary infection present of lesions not responding to home treatment

Emergency

Cross Reference   Fungal Infections

KIDNEY STONES (Renal Calculi)

An abnormal concretion occurring within the kidney

Etiology
Excessive excretion of relatively insoluble urinary constituents (calcium, oxalate, cystine, uric acid); physical changes in urine; nucleus for stone formation (e.g., bits of necrotic tissue, clumps of bacteria); congenital or acquired deformities of the kidneys

Assessment
Usual symptoms include flank pain and colic, nausea, vomiting, abdominal distention, hematuria, chills, fever; possible bladder irritability. Differentiate from acute pyelonephritis, infarction of the kidney. Check for degree of pain (males describe this as "worst pain of my life"). Is pain relieved with pain meds? History of similar problem? Check for amount of vomiting, possible dehydration.

Treatment/ Teaching
Analgesics as ordered. Fluids when pain is controlled. Strain urine. Nausea and vomiting interventions prn.

Refer to MD
If no relief with pain medications; dysuria, anuria, or hematuria

Emergency
Severe pain

Cross Reference
Abdominal Pain; Blood in Urine; Dehydration; Pain in Side; Nausea and Vomiting; Urine, Dark-Colored; Urine, Decreased Output or Stream; Voiding Difficulty

A wound, usually linear, into the skin

Etiology Trauma

Assessment Determine if any loss of motor or sensory function, how the injury occurred, site, depth and length of laceration, presence of active bleeding.

Treatment/ Teaching Stop bleeding with direct pressure. Keep wound clean; wash well with soap and water, rinse off, apply antibiotic ointment (Bacitracin or Polysporin) 3 times a day for 3 to 4 days. Apply dressing prn. Check for current tetanus immunization. If previous immunization but no booster in past 5 years, refer to MD or Health Department within 72 hours of injury for booster. If no previous immunization, refer to MD immediately. Be seen by MD within 4 to 6 hours of injury if suturing required (i.e., if wound is on face, or is deep and edges do not come together). For lacerations within mouth, have client use ice in mouth to stop bleeding; rinse mouth with salt water after eating (no suturing unless laceration comes through to outside or unless tongue is severely lacerated or deeper tissue involved). Watch all lacerations for signs of infection.

Refer to MD If unable to stop bleeding, if suturing and/or tetanus immunization required, if wound infection develops; refer immediately if no previous tetanus immunization.

Emergency Extensive laceration, severed digit or tendon

Cross Reference Bites, Animal and Human (Peds); Tetanus Immunization (Peds); Wound Infection

A state of inaction or indifference; a subjective feeling associated with inactivity and decreased energy

Etiology Illness, depression, unknown causes

Assessment A certain amount of lethargy follows or accompanies almost every clinical disturbance. Often there is no relationship to either weakness or fatigue. Rely on history and ancillary symptoms. Determine the degree of lethargy present: what is the client's activity level? level of responsiveness?

Treatment/ Teaching Mild lethargy is a normal component of many illnesses. Rest and decrease activity level until illness is over.

Refer to MD For evaluation of prolonged lethargy, or if associated with ancillary symptoms requiring evaluation and treatment, for counseling if associated with symptoms of depression

Emergency

Cross Reference Depression, Drowsiness, Fatigue, Mononucleosis

Parasitic infestation of skin, scalp, trunk, or pubic areas

Etiology   Pubic, body, or head louse. The head louse is transmitted through shared clothing and brushes, the body louse by bedding or clothing, and the pubic louse from person-to-person, frequently on clothing, bedding, or towels.

Assessment   Usual symptoms include itching with excoriation, eggs (nits) on hair shafts, lice on skin or clothes. R/o scabies, seborrheic dermatitis of the scalp.

Treatment/ Teaching   No sharing of bedding, clothing, brushes, towels. In the past, Kwell (shampoo and lotion) has been the drug of choice for treatment of lice; however, this drug may have systemic side effects. RID and A-200 Pyrinate are equally effective against lice and can be safely used by all individuals except those suffering from ragweed allergy (hay fever). Refer to Antiparasytics in Pediatric Doses of Commonly Used Medications for appropriate recommendations.

Scalp: Apply medication thoroughly. After thorough rinsing, the hair should be cleaned with a fine-toothed comb to remove nit shells. Nits are difficult to remove. A white vinegar/water solution (1:1) is sometimes useful as a hair rinse to aid in removal of nits. Disinfect combs and brushes by washing. Launder clothing, caps, linens.

Body: May only need to wash with soap and water and apply topical antipruritic lotions. Alternatively, lice may be eliminated by dusting with 1% malathion powder or 10% DDT powder. Lice in clothing (usually found in seams) may be killed by boiling, followed by ironing the seams, dry cleaning, or application of dry heat at 140° for 20 minutes.

Pubic: Treatment may be repeated in 7 days prn. Treat all family members showing symptoms. Wash clothing, linens, and towels in very hot water or dry clean.

Other: Pets may be vectors and should be bathed with appropriate medicated shampoo. Spray inanimate objects not able to be washed (mattress, carpet, furniture); vacuum all and throw out disposable bag. Lice can live without host for 5 to 10 days.

Refer to MD   For diagnosis of scabies or body lice, prn for recurring infection or other complications; also refer for any questions re the use of Kwell, i.e., in debilitated, elderly, or newborn clients.

Emergency

Cross Reference   Itching, Pediatric Doses of Commonly Used Medications (Antiparasitics), Scabies

Cracks or sores on the lips

Etiology Exposure to cold, dry weather; bacterial or viral infections

Assessment Rely on history and ancillary symptoms.

Treatment/ Teaching A&D Ointment, Vaseline, or Chapstick if lesions are due to exposure to cold, dry weather, or URI.

Refer to MD If lesions not healing with home treatment, or if spreading and symptoms increasing

Emergency

Cross Reference Cold Sore; Herpes Simplex; Impetigo

Inflammation of the meninges covering the brain and spinal cord

Etiology Bacteria or virus

Assessment Usual symptoms include fever, headache, vomiting; possible confusion, delirium, convulsions; petechial rash of skin and mucous membranes; back and neck stiffness, abdominal and extremity pain. Symptoms may follow a URI. Check for severity of headache, degree of fever, stiffness of neck, presence of projectile vomiting, degree of activity, state of alertness.

Treatment/ Teaching Persons with close contact to a client with bacterial meningitis need prophylactic antibiotic therapy.

Refer to MD If symptoms suspect, but inconclusive and mild

Emergency Severe symptoms

Cross Reference Convulsions, Fever, Headache, Nausea and Vomiting, Neck Pain, Petechiae, Rash

A severe, rapidly progressive, bacterial infection of the blood stream

Etiology Neisseria Meningitidis

Assessment Onset is usually sudden with fever, chills, vomiting, weakness; often associated with meningitis. A petechial skin rash may develop rapidly. The course of the septicemic form is rapid, ending in death if therapy not instituted early.

Treatment/ Teaching Contacts should be treated. Contact MD same day as exposure.

Refer to MD For treatment of contacts

Emergency If severely ill with or without petechial rash

Cross Reference Meningitis, Petechiae

Symptoms that may accompany the cessation of menstruation

Etiology   Declining ovarian function

Assessment   Amenorrhea is frequently preceded by irregular menstrual periods (i.e., irregular intervals and sometimes heavier flow), hot flashes, and feelings of tension—especially fullness in head. Weight gain and nervous instability with depression, exhilaration, or lassitude are often present. Changes in sexual interest, painful breasts, and various aches and "rheumatic pains" may occur. Bladder irritation is common. R/o anxiety states and depression, organic causes of back pain.

Treatment/ Teaching   Recognize that depression, mood swings, irregular flow are normal responses to menopause. Menopausal support groups may be available. Hormonal therapy (per MD) may decrease some of the symptoms.

Refer to MD   For evaluation of troublesome symptoms

Emergency

Cross Reference   Amenorrhea

Excessive, regular, monthly menstrual flow

Etiology Usually due to local lesions (i.e., uterine myomas, endometrial polyps), salpingitis, or endometritis

Assessment The heavy flow is cyclical, but may or may not be of normal length. Check if client on anticoagulant therapy or chemotherapy. Check for possible pregnancy, fever, and presence of IUD. R/o threatened abortion, displaced IUD.

Treatment/ Teaching Bedrest to attempt to reduce flow

Refer to MD For management of chronic problem; be seen if saturating 1 pad in less than 2 hours or if flowing more heavily than normal

Emergency Hemorrhage and/or shock

Cross Reference Abortion, Dysmenorrhea, Fatigue, Shock

Etiology

Assessment

**Treatment/
Teaching**

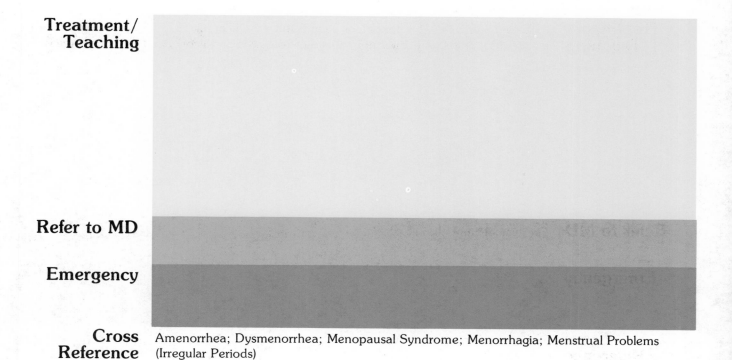

Refer to MD

Emergency

**Cross
Reference**   Amenorrhea; Dysmenorrhea; Menopausal Syndrome; Menorrhagia; Menstrual Problems
(Irregular Periods)

Menstrual periods occurring less often than the usual monthly cycle

Etiology Pregnancy, menarche, menopause, endocrine disorder, systemic problems, absence of ovulation, vigorous athletic training (e.g., marathon running)

Assessment R/o pregnancy.

**Treatment/
Teaching** Following menarche, it is normal for periods to be irregular for 12 to 40 cycles. If related to menopause, reassure that it is normal and caution woman to continue birth control measures.

Refer to MD For evaluation of chronic problem

Emergency

**Cross
Reference** Pregnancy, Menopausal Syndrome

Paroxysmal attacks of headache often preceded by psychologic or visual disturbances and sometimes followed by drowsiness

Etiology   Vascular changes

Assessment   Characteristically, a migraine is preceded by a prodrome consisting of visual abnormalities or other sensory-motor dysfunctions on the side of the body opposite to that of the headache. Prodrome may be absent in some cases. The headache is usually unilateral, throbbing, and may be accompanied by nausea and vomiting as pain becomes intense. Migraine in the eye will produce weird visual disturbances (e.g., "flashing lights"). They occur in about 8% of the population and are more frequent in women than men.

Treatment/ Teaching   Rest in dark, quiet room; sit up until medication begins to reduce pain, then lie down. Heat to neck. Medications as prescribed to help prevent headache and/or to provide pain relief.

Refer to MD   If unable to get relief with medications and home treatment, or for disturbing visual distortions

Emergency

Cross Reference   Headache

Circumscribed pigmented macules, papules, or nodules comprised of clusters of nevus cells; may be present at birth or develop later

Etiology Nevus cells

Assessment Usually benign; almost everyone has at least a few of these lesions. Commonly appear in childhood and tend to undergo spontaneous fibrosis in old age.

Treatment/ Teaching Watch for change in size, color, or development of tenderness, itching, or bleeding. Moles on belt-, bra-, collar-lines may need to be removed.

Refer to MD If above symptoms (changes) develop; for evaluation/removal

Emergency

Cross Reference

Acute, infectious disease (usually benign) of the body characterized by an abnormally large number of monocytes in the blood

Etiology   Epstein-Barr (EB) herpes virus

Assessment   Usual symptoms include fever, sore throat, malaise, lymphadenopathy, occasional maculopapular rash. Usually occurs between ages of 10 to 35, either in epidemic or sporadic cases. Mode of transmission probably droplet. Incubation period usually 5 to 15 days. In an uncomplicated case, fever disappears in 10 days; lymphadenopathy and splenomegaly in 4 weeks. Sometimes illness lingers 2 to 3 months. R/o streptococcal tonsillitis, diphtheria, rubella, hepatitis.

Treatment/ Teaching   ASA every 4 hours prn fever, sore throat. Do not give acetaminophen (excreted by the liver, which is already compromised). Saline gargles. Fluids. Bedrest during acute phase. Support and reassurance because of frequent feeling of lassitude and duration of symptoms.

Refer to MD   For diagnosis, treatment of complications (e.g., secondary throat infections, hepatitis, CNS involvement, Guillain-Barré syndrome, pulmonary involvement)

Emergency   Evidence of ruptured spleen

Cross Reference   Fever, Lethargy, Rash, Saline Gargles (Glossary), Sore Throat, Swollen Glands

MORNING SICKNESS

Nausea and vomiting due to pregnancy

Etiology   Unknown; may be caused by high levels of estrogen and HCG

Assessment   Usual onset is during the 5th to 6th week of pregnancy, persisting until the 14th to 16th week. Symptoms are usually most severe in the mornings. R/o other causes of vomiting.

Treatment/ Teaching   Reassure that about 50% of pregnant women (usually primiparas) complain of nausea and vomiting during pregnancy. Try dry foods at frequent intervals, (e.g., soda crackers, dry toast). Restrict fats, odorous foods, spiced dishes, and items that do not appeal to the client. Try sipping coke syrup or sucking on hard candy. Discontinue smoking.

Refer to MD   For medication to control nausea and vomiting, or if vomiting is excessive

Emergency

Cross Reference   Nausea and Vomiting; Pregnancy, Minor Discomforts Of

An acute, contagious, febrile condition characterized by inflammation of the salivary glands

Etiology

Virus

Assessment

Tender parotid swelling is the most common physical finding. Fever and malaise are variable. Pain and swelling of one or both (75%) of the parotids or other salivary glands occurs, usually in succession, 1 to 3 days apart. Occasionally, 1 gland will subside completely before others become involved. Orchitis occurs in 25% of men. Headache and lethargy suggest meningoencephalitis. High fever usually accompanies orchitis or meningoencephalitis. Upper abdominal pain and nausea and vomiting suggest pancreatitis. Lower abdominal pain in females suggests oophoritis. R/o calculi in parotid ducts, iodine reaction, or abscess. Differentiate swelling of the parotid gland from inflammation of the lymph nodes located more posteriorly and inferiorly than the parotid.

Treatment/ Teaching

Spread by respiratory droplets; isolate client until swelling subsides; bedrest while febrile; fluids; analgesics for discomfort, antipyretics for fever; soft diet; ice collar or ice pack prn discomfort. Immunization is available but may not be helpful if exposure has already occurred.

Refer to MD

For males exposed to mumps with no history of having them; for diagnosis

Emergency

Cross Reference

Fever, Ice Pack and Ice Collar (Glossary), Immunization Information, Swelling (Peds)

MUSCLE PAIN OR SPASM

Inflammation or injury of skeletal muscle causing pain and/or spasm

Etiology Viral illness, local injury

Assessment Rely on history and ancillary symptoms. Determine location, onset, frequency, intensity, extent of mobility and pain, any loss of motor or sensory function, things that exacerbate or relieve it, radiation, history of similar pain.

Treatment/ Teaching Apply ice or heat locally to reduce spasm and pain. ASA prn pain (acetaminophen if viral etiolgy suspected). Gentle massage often helpful (frozen juice can wrapped in light towel and rolled over area in spasm). Bed rest and/or limited activity until spasm subsides. Use correct body mechanics when lifting heavy objects.

Refer to MD If no relief with home treatment

Emergency

Cross Reference Back Pain, Ice Massage (Glossary), Neck Pain, Strain

Lack of functional strength of skeletal muscles

Etiology   Viral infection, CVA, brain tumor, chronic illness, medication, Guillain-Barré syndrome

Assessment   Rely on history and ancillary symptoms.

Treatment/ Teaching   Range-of-motion and specific muscle-strengthening exercises if related to aftermath of CVA.

Refer to MD   For evaluation and treatment if cause unknown and client not extremely incapacitated

Emergency   Client totally incapacitated; respiratory muscle weakness apparent (i.e., severe dyspnea)

Cross Reference   Guillain-Barré Syndrome, Stroke

Damage to a portion of the heart muscle due to myocardial ischemia

Etiology Usually coronary artery occlusion

Assessment 80% of clients with MI have history of angina. Pain may begin during rest or activity, is more severe than pain of angina. It builds up steadily, rapidly, or in waves to maximum intensity in space of few minutes or longer. Nitroglycerin has little effect. Pain often unbearable and may last for hours if unrelieved by narcotics; may radiate to shoulder, jaw, arms. Diaphoresis is high index of probability for MI. Client feels weak, apprehensive, prefers not to lie quietly. Other signs and symptoms include lightheadedness, syncope, dyspnea, orthopnea, cough, wheezing, nausea and vomiting, heartburn, or abdominal pain. May have post-MI symptoms (i.e., pericarditis, fever, chills).

Treatment/ Teaching Try to keep client quiet and in position of comfort while emergency aid is en route.

Refer to MD Arrange emergency transportation to hospital

Emergency Arrange emergency transportation to hospital

Cross Reference Chest Pain, Coma, Cyanosis, Fainting, Heartburn, Indigestion, Nausea and Vomiting, Shock

Suppurative inflammation around a fingernail

Etiology   Usually staphylococcus; may be fungus, virus, or yeast

Assessment   Infection may superficially follow the nail margin, or may extend beneath the nail, suppurate, and cause pain. Infection may be acute, subacute, or chronic. Fungal infections are not so painful and cause a serous drainage. Bacterial infection appears more inflamed with purulent drainage.

Treatment/ Teaching   Hot soaks if infection appears bacterial (contraindicated for fungal infection).

Refer to MD   If no improvement with hot soaks, or needs incision and drainage (often the only action that will relieve throbbing pain)

Emergency   Red streak up arm (lymphangitis)

Cross Reference

Sensation of pressure, blockage, or fullness in nasal passages, with or without nasal discharge and pain

Etiology URI, sinus infection or congestion, allergies, foreign body

Assessment Rely on history and ancillary symptoms.

Treatment/ Teaching Decongestant (e.g., Sudafed, Chlortrimeton, Coricidin D). Vaporizer. Clear fluids; avoid dairy products. Elevate head. Saline nose drops. Vasoconstricting nose drops (e.g., Neo-Synephrine or Afrin); use nose drops only 5 days at a time, then discontinue.

Refer to MD If no relief with home treatment, if foreign body or infection suspected (i.e., purulent yellow or green discharge and fever); for evaluation of possible allergy

Emergency

Cross Reference Cold Symptoms, Hay Fever, Saline Nose Drops (Glossary), Sinus Congestion, Sinus Infection, Upper Respiratory Infection

Feeling of queasiness or actual evacuation of stomach contents

Etiology Irritation, inflammation, or mechanical disturbance at any level of GI tract due to organic or functional disorders (e.g., cholecystitis, inner ear disturbances, side or toxic effects of drugs, central emetics, toxins, increased intracranial pressure, cerebral hypoxia due to cerebral ischemia or hemorrhage, psychologic factors, pregnancy)

Assessment Rely on history and ancillary symptoms. Determine amount and frequency of vomiting, presence of projectile vomiting, onset and duration, presence or absence of signs of dehydration.

Treatment/ Teaching Nothing PO for 2 to 3 hours. If vomiting subsides, start sips of water (1 tsp every 10 minutes for 30 minutes). If fluid retained, increase amount of clear fluid. May use flat 7-Up, Gatorade, tea, broth. Diet as tolerated when clear fluids can be retained. Watch urine output as indicator of dehydration.

Refer to MD For intractable vomiting unrelieved by home treatment; if due to head injury; if associated with other serious symptoms; if dehydration probable

Emergency Emesis of large amounts of blood, extreme pain, or life-threatening symptoms

Cross Reference Anorexia; Appendicitis; Congestive Heart Failure; Dehydration; Ear Infection; Food Poisoning; Gall Bladder Colic; Gastroenteritis; Head Injury; Hepatitis; Influenza; Kidney Stones; Meningitis; Morning Sickness; Myocardial Infarction; Obstruction; Salmonella Infection; Stroke; Toxic Shock Syndrome; Ulcer, Duodenal and Gastric; Urinary Tract Infection

Discomfort in posterior cervical area

Etiology   Injury, muscle spasm, pinched nerve, meningitis

Assessment   Rely on history and ancillary symptoms. Assess onset, frequency, location, character of pain, things that exacerbate or relieve it, radiation, history of similar pain.

Treatment/ Teaching   **Muscle spasm/pinched nerve:** Rest. Ice pack or heat to area, ASA, muscle relaxant (if client already has that available). Make cervical collar with bath towel to reduce neck muscle use.

Refer to MD   For management of chronic problem or evaluation of neck injury, if symptoms suspicious of meningitis but are inconclusive and mild

Emergency   Severe pain, associated paralysis, if client extremely ill with suspected meningitis

Cross Reference   Ice Pack (Glossary), Meningitis, Muscle Pain or Spasm, Strain

Pruritic or stinging rash following contact with nettles plant

Etiology   Contact with nettles plant

Assessment   Rash appears on body surface exposed to plant, develops quickly after exposure.

Treatment/ Teaching   Cold packs or compresses. Calamine lotion to lesions. ASA to reduce pain and/or itching. Oral antihistamines prn itching (e.g., CTM, Benadryl). Avoid further contact with plant. Underside of bracken fern, which usually grows next to nettles, rubbed on site is natural antidote.

Refer to MD   If secondary infection develops or if resolution does not follow usual course (i.e., if rash spreads or systemic allergic symptoms develop)

Emergency

Cross Reference   Dermatitis, Contact

Awakening to pass urine during the night

Etiology   Urinary tract infection, prostatitis, benign prostatic hypertrophy, urinary retention, excessive fluid intake, pregnancy, diuretics, excretion of edema fluid accumulated during the day, increased renal perfusion in the recumbent position, diabetes mellitus, diabetes insipidus

Assessment   Rely on history and ancillary symptoms.

Treatment/ Teaching   Avoid tea, coffee, alcohol, spices if problem due to pregnancy. Avoid drinking fluids close to bedtime. Take prescribed diuretics in morning.

Refer to MD   For evaluation if problem persists and/or evidence of infection

Emergency

Cross Reference   Pregnancy, Minor Discomforts Of; Prostatitis; Urinary Tract Infection

Bleeding from the nose

Etiology External trauma, nose picking, nasal infection, drying of nasal mucosa, systemic illness

Assessment Rely on history. R/o blood dyscrasias, hypertension, hemorrhagic disease, nasal tumors, measles, rheumatic fever (if nosebleeds recurrent or profuse without obvious cause).

Treatment/ Teaching Sit up and blow clots out gently. Pinch nose, grasping entire lower portion of nose below boney part, and hold for 10 minutes (by the clock). Breathe and spit through mouth. May use Neo-Synephrine pledget in nose as vasoconstrictor to slow bleeding. Ice pack to bridge of nose.

Refer to MD If nosebleeds are recurrent and/or severe, if bleeding not stopped with home treatment in 10 minutes

Emergency Uncontrolled epistaxsis

Cross Reference Nose, Broken

Fracture of the nasal bone

Etiology   Usually trauma

Assessment   R/o head injury. Check for malalignment of nose, free flow of air from both nostrils, obstruction.

Treatment/ Teaching   Treat for nose bleed prn. Ice pack to reduce swelling. Expect some discoloration on nose and possibly around eyes. Watch for signs of head injury.

Refer to MD   For evaluation of fracture; be seen within 6 to 8 hours to check for septal hematoma, which, although rare, must be drained; usually not seen for manipulation until edema has decreased (about 3 days)

Emergency   Uncontrolled epistaxsis, evidence of head injury

Cross Reference   Fractures or Dislocations, Head Injury, Ice Pack (Glossary), Nosebleed

A sensory abnormality resulting in a distortion or absence of response to tactile or painful stimuli

Etiology Compression, ischemia, trauma, infection, vascular or metabolic disease, neoplasms, exposure to heavy metals

Assessment Determine degree of numbness and location. Check for signs of impaired circulation (i.e., skin is cool or cold to touch, pale, or cyanotic), evidence of decreased muscle function. Rely on history and ancillary symptoms.

Treatment/ Teaching Protect numb area (may be more likely to be injured because of decreased sensation).

Refer to MD For evaluation of chronic problem; if evidence of mild to moderate circulatory impairment; for evaluation of ancillary symptoms

Emergency Rapidly progressing numbness and/or evidence of serious circulatory impairment

Cross Reference Bell's Palsy, Cast Care, Fractures or Dislocations, Guillain-Barré Syndrome, Hyperventilation, Shingles, Stroke

Blockage of the intestinal tract due to mechanical factors or failure of peristalsis

Etiology Hernia, adhesions, volvulus, tumor, stricture, fecal impaction, foreign body, inflammation of intestinal wall; peristaltic failure may follow surgery or occur during many severe acute diseases such as pneumonia and MI, or following trauma (e.g., compression fracture of vertebra).

Assessment Crampy, intermittent, or severe steady pain; vomiting that may resemble dilute feces in odor and appearance, abdominal distension, dehydration. Early mechanical obstruction may be confused with gastroenteritis; continued vomiting and abdominal pain usually suggest that an obstruction, not a self-limiting gastroenteritis, is the problem.

Treatment/ Teaching Heat to abdomen for 20 minutes. Nausea and vomiting protocol (see cross reference card).

Refer to MD For evaluation and diagnosis, if symptoms unresolved with home treatment, or dehydration present

Emergency Severe abdominal pain, signs of internal hemorrhage

Cross Reference Abdominal Pain, Nausea and Vomiting

Medication taken in excess of therapeutic dose

Etiology   Intentional, accidental

Assessment   Rely on history and ancillary symptoms. Ask what drug was taken, how it was taken, time it was taken, how much was taken, how much the client weighs.

Treatment/ Teaching   Encourage an understanding, responsible person to stay with the client. Ipecac as emetic if appropriate (per Poison Control guidelines). Contact Poison Control Center for specific instructions, signs to watch for. Contact mental health unit if appropriate.

Poison Control Center:

Refer to MD   For evaluation and follow-up prn

Emergency   Semi-comatose, comatose; respiratory distress; highly toxic material ingested

Cross Reference   Aspirin Overdose, Coma, Fainting, Ipecac Protocol (Peds), Suicide

OVERWEIGHT (Obesity)

Weight increase of over 10% above normal for age, sex, body type

Etiology Intake of more calories than are required for energy metabolism

Assessment R/o endocrine and metabolic disorders (relatively rare), fluid retention.

Treatment/ Teaching Diet is most important factor in management of obesity. An intake of 500 calories per day less than required should lead to an average weight loss of approximately 0.5 kg (1 lb) a week. A daily intake of 800 to 1200 calories is satisfactory for modest reducing diet. Increased physical activity important in long-range weight-reducing efforts. Support groups such as Weight Watchers and Overeaters Anonymous are often helpful.

Weight Watchers: _____

Overeaters Anonymous: _____

Refer to MD For specific diet, exercise instructions, and follow-up

Emergency

Cross Reference

Information about sources of oxygen

Etiology

Assessment

Treatment/ Teaching

Need verbal order from MD. Oxygen is available in cylinders and liquid form 24 hours a day through any of the following companies (write in for your area):

_____

_____

_____

The respiratory therapy department located in a local hospital can usually make all necessary arrangements for home oxygen on a 24-hour basis. Reinforce O_2 precautions (i.e., no smoking); offer guidelines for flow adjustment and client positioning.

Refer to MD

Emergency

Cross Reference

Emphysema

Discomfort in flank area between ribs and hip

Etiology   UTI, renal calculi, musculoskeletal pain, injury, aneurysm

Assessment   Determine onset, frequency, radiation, intensity of pain; things that exacerbate or relieve it; areas of localized tenderness; presence of fever; visible injury to area; urinary symptoms; other ancillary symptoms.

Treatment/ Teaching   For pain that is muscular in nature, use local heat, rest. Analgesics; may need narcotics for pain of renal calculi.

Refer to MD   For evaluation and treatment of UTI, injury, or renal calculi pain

Emergency   Severe, incapacitating pain

Cross Reference   Aneurysm, Ruptured Aortic; Kidney Stones; Urinary Tract Infection

Rapid, forceful beating of the heart of which the client is conscious

Etiology

Assessment

**Treatment/
Teaching**

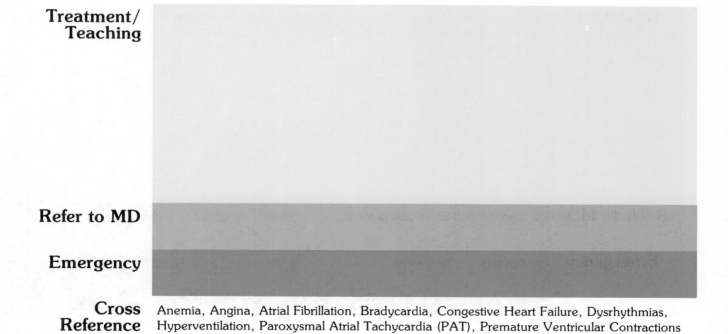

Refer to MD

Emergency

**Cross
Reference** Anemia, Angina, Atrial Fibrillation, Bradycardia, Congestive Heart Failure, Dysrhythmias, Hyperventilation, Paroxysmal Atrial Tachycardia (PAT), Premature Ventricular Contractions (PVCs)

Complete or incomplete loss of nervous function to part(s) of the body

Etiology CVA, injury to affected part, hysteria, tick-bite paralysis, multiple sclerosis, Bell's palsy, Guillain-Barré syndrome, myasthenia gravis, lesions in CNS

Assessment Rely on history and ancillary symptoms.

Treatment/ Teaching Range-of-motion or gradually increasing exercise of paralyzed part if appropriate (i.e., following CVA). Good skin care and positioning to prevent decubiti and contractures. Turn client frequently.

Refer to MD For management of chronic problem

Emergency Sudden onset of symptoms

Cross Reference Bell's Palsy; Guillain-Barré Syndrome; Stroke; Ulcer, Decubitus

Heart rate suddenly increases to 140 or more/minute; role of normal pacemaker is displaced

Etiology   Most commonly occurs in young clients with normal hearts; inflammatory or degenerative myocardial disease, cardiac failure from any cause; anxiety, fatigue, or disturbed psychologic states

Assessment   Attacks begin and end abruptly and may last several hours. Heart rate may be 140 to 240/minute (usually 170 to 220) and is perfectly regular. Exercise, change of position, breath-holding have no effect. Clients are asymptomatic except for awareness of rapid heart action unless underlying heart disease present.

Treatment/ Teaching   If client feels all right and has no chest pain, is not lightheaded, and heart rate is less than 150, regular, and strong, reassure that the episode is usually transient, should cause no permanent harm, and should stop in 10 to 20 minutes. It may be terminated by having the client take a deep breath and bear down as if straining to have a bowel movement (Valsalva's maneuver). Carotid massage (**one side at a time**) may be recommended in younger clients only (under 40-years-old). Some clients have instructions to take Inderal or Valium. Discontinue caffeine.

Refer to MD   For evaluation if attacks are frequent and/or long lasting

Emergency   Heart rate over 150 but client feels weak or other cardiac symptoms present (angina or congestive heart symptoms)

Cross Reference   Dysrhythmias

Drainage from the penis

Etiology   Venereal disease, nonspecific urethritis

Assessment

Treatment/ Teaching   Client should be seen same day for diagnosis. No sexual activity until diagnosis established.

Refer to MD   For diagnosis and treatment

Emergency

Cross Reference   Gonorrhea

A sore on the penis

Etiology   Venereal disease, venereal warts, injury, herpes, monilia, bacterial infection

Assessment Rely on history and ancillary symptoms.

Treatment/ Determine exposure to venereal disease if possible. Use condom during intercourse if lesions
Teaching   due to venereal disease.

Refer to MD For evaluation and treatment

Emergency

Cross   Herpes, Genital; Venereal Warts; Syphilis
Reference

Small hemorrhagic spots on the skin

Etiology Idiopathic thrombocytopenic purpura, meningitis, meningococcemia, leukemia, trauma, side effect of drugs, prolonged bleeding, bite from brown recluse spider, blood dyscrasias

Assessment Rely on history and ancillary symptoms.

Treatment/ Teaching

Refer to MD If diagnosis previously established and no additional symptoms are occurring; if new case

Emergency Sudden onset of symptoms

Cross Reference Meningitis, Meningococcemia, Spider Bites

Infection of the pelvic organs

Etiology   Usually bacteria (gonococci, streptococci, or mixed bacterial flora)

Assessment   Usual symptoms include leukorrhea; severe cramplike, nonradiating, lower abdominal pain; chills; moderately high, intermittent fever; abnormal menstruation or abortion; painful intercourse. May be acute or chronic. R/o acute appendicitis, ectopic pregnancy, salpingitis (usually unilateral, may be associated with use of an IUD).

**Treatment/
Teaching**

Refer to MD   For evaluation and treatment

Emergency

**Cross
Reference**   Abdominal Pain, Appendicitis, Ectopic Pregnancy

PIMPLES (Papules)

Small, circumscribed, erythematous, elevations of the skin

Etiology   Blocked sebaceous gland, bacteria

Assessment

Treatment/   Do not squeeze. Keep area clean; use medicated soap and water (Fostex and Oxy 5 are good
Teaching   cleansers). Hot pack prn to form pustules.

Refer to MD   If area becomes more infected (i.e., streaking, swelling, and inflammation), especially on face
with possibility of cellulitis; for specific medications; if problem is not resolving; for further
evaluation

Emergency   Signs of rapidly developing cellulitis, especially facial lesions above the lip line

Cross   Acne, Boil, Cellulitis, Erysipelas
Reference

Etiology

Assessment

**Treatment/
Teaching**

Refer to MD

Emergency

**Cross
Reference**   Conjunctivitis

PINWORMS (Enterobiasis)

Infestation of bowel with short, spindle-shaped worms

Etiology   Enterobius vermicularis

Assessment   Humans are only host for the parasite. Children are affected more commonly than adults. Usual symptoms include perianal pruritis (usually nocturnal) associated with insomnia and restlessness, vague gastrointestinal symptoms, appearance of worms and larvae around rectal opening.

Treatment/ Teaching   Careful hand washing after defecation and before meals. Fingernails trimmed close and kept clean. Wash infected bed linen and underwear in hot soap and water. Zinc oxide to perianal area to reduce itching and help interrupt worm's life cycle (prevents female from getting out of rectum to lay eggs). Drug of choice is Vermox; treat just the symptomatic members of the family; no systemic treatment for anyone under 2 years of age or pregnant.

Refer to MD   For verification of diagnosis and follow-up if symptoms return; if urinary symptoms present and infection suspected

Emergency

Cross Reference   Itching, Pinworms (Peds), Worms

Condition in which the placenta is implanted low in the uterus completely or partially covering the internal os of the cervix.

Etiology   None known

Assessment   Usual symptoms include sudden, painless, scant or profuse bleeding in late pregnancy.

Treatment/ Teaching   Arrange for emergency transportation to the hospital

Refer to MD

Emergency   Uterine hemorrhage; emergency transportation to hospital (immediate care may be required, including Cesarean section)

Cross Reference   Vaginal Hemorrhage

Inflammation of the pleura

Etiology   Usually secondary to pulmonary disease (pneumonia, pulmonary infarction, neoplasm)

Assessment   Chest pain is greatest with inspiration. Pain is minimal or absent when breath is held or when ribs are splinted. Clients may have decreased motion of the chest and shallow "grunting" respirations. Onset is sudden. Fever and malaise almost always present. Short, painful, non-productive cough.

Treatment/ Teaching   Analgesics (ASA or Acetaminophen) prn pain. Evaluate for possible cardiac problems and respiratory distress. Heat to involved area.

Refer to MD   For evaluation of underlying disease and management of pain

Emergency

Cross Reference   Chest Pain, Cold Symptoms, Pulmonary Embolus, Upper Respiratory Infection

An acute infection of the alveolar spaces of the lung

Etiology   Bacteria, virus, tubercle bacillus, rickettsia, fungus, aspiration

Assessment   Bacterial infection often preceded by URI; sudden onset of shaking, chills, fever, chest pain, and cough with rust-colored sputum. Chest pain usually exaggerated by coughing; may be referred to shoulder, abdomen, or flank. Client appears very ill, marked increase in respiratory rate without orthopnea; often lies on affected side to splint the chest.

Treatment/ Teaching   Bed rest during acute phase; clear fluids; cough expectorant and/or suppressant (e.g., Benylin, Robitussin); elevate head; vaporizer or steamy bathroom. ASA for fever (acetaminophen if viral etiology is suspected). Heat to chest for pain; may require narcotic analgesic for relief.

Refer to MD   For diagnosis, treatment, evaluation; to check for aspirated foreign body, respiratory status (need for oxygen), and/or hospitalization

Emergency   Severe dyspnea, pulmonary edema, shock

Cross Reference   Breathing Difficulty, Cold Symptoms, Cough, Fever, Influenza, Pulmonary Edema, Shock, Upper Respiratory Infection

Free air in the pleural cavity between chest wall and lung

Etiology   Unknown; may be secondary to injury or pulmonary disease

Assessment   Sudden onset of chest pain referred to shoulder or arm on involved side; associated with dyspnea, decreased chest motion, decreased breath and voice sounds on involved side.

Treatment/ Teaching   Close chest wound, if present, with any available means (bandage, handkerchief, shirt, etc.) **THIS IS AN EMERGENCY!!!** Arrange for emergency transportation to hospital.

Refer to MD

Emergency   Emergency transportation to hospital

Cross Reference   Chest Pain, Cyanosis

Ingestion of a poisonous substance or medication in an excessive dose

Etiology Accidental or intentional

Assessment Rely on history of ingestion and presence of symptoms. Determine what was ingested, time of ingestion, weight of client, presence of symptoms, quantity of substance ingested.

**Treatment/
Teaching** Contact Poison Control Center for direction regarding proper handling of the situation. If Ipecac is given, recontact client or client's family in 20 to 25 minutes to determine if vomiting occurred after Ipecac was administered. Identify a responsible person to stay with the client to monitor symptoms and/or to transport to medical facility.

Poison Control Center: _____

Refer to MD If advised by Poison Control or if Ipecac not effective in inducing vomiting

Emergency Toxic symptoms, potential life-threatening situation

**Cross
Reference** Aspirin Overdose, Cyanosis, Ipecac Protocol (Peds), Overdose

A contact dermatitis

Etiology   Contact with poison oak or poison ivy

Assessment   Common sites are usually on exposed areas of skin; often linear from brushing contact with allergen. Reaction includes erythematous macules, papules, and vesicles; area often hot and swollen with exudation, crusting, and secondary infection. Asymmetric distribution and history of contact help establish diagnosis.

Treatment/ Teaching   Bathe in cool water, cool compresses. Calamine lotion (no Caladryl, Nupercainal, or Lidocaine ointment). Oral antihistamines (e.g., Benedryl) may reduce itching. Wash all clothing worn during contact.

Refer to MD   If lesions are widespread

Emergency

Cross Reference   Dermatitis, Contact

Temporary depressive state that occurs shortly after the birth of a baby

Etiology Reaction by the new mother to the sudden emotional and physical care responsibilities of a newborn

Assessment In the early postpartum period (usually within the 1st week), the new mother will experience periods of discouragement and a feeling of depression as she attempts to cope with the drudgery, personal sacrifice, fatigue, and the responsibility she must accept for the care of a completely dependent infant. R/o psychosis, schizophrenia, or other more severe psychiatric disorders.

Treatment/ Teaching Reassurance and support for the mother; assure her that she is experiencing a normal reaction that usually subsides. Determine the need for visiting nurse referral and more intensive counseling.

Refer to MD For further counseling or evaluation of a more severe psychiatric problem

Emergency

Cross Reference Depression

Toxemia of pregnancy

Etiology Unknown; predisposing factors include malnutrition, vascular and renal disease, sodium retention, multiple pregnancy

Assessment Usually seen in the last trimester of pregnancy. Preeclampsia denotes nonconvulsive form. Symptoms include headaches, hypertension, proteinuria, and edema. Eclampsia indicates development of convulsions and coma. Symptoms include headache, vertigo, irritability, convulsions, coma, partial or complete blindness, nausea, vomiting, epigastric pain, elevated blood pressure, edema, oliguria, anuria.

Treatment/ Teaching If already diagnosed and home treatment indicated: bedrest; lie on left side. Monitor intake and output; fluids (8 to 12 glasses/day). Frequent blood pressure readings. Sodium restriction. Daily urine protein determinations. Sedatives as prescribed.

Refer to MD For diagnosis and treatment; evaluation of need for hospitalization if not responding to home treatment

Emergency Convulsions, coma, vision problems, anuria, oliguria

Cross Reference

Usual discomforts during normal pregnancy

Etiology   Physiologic changes due to pregnancy

Assessment   Rely on history and ancillary symptoms.

Treatment/ Teaching

Abdominal discomfort/pressure (due to weight of uterus on pelvic supports): Frequent rest periods; use maternity girdle for support.

Round ligament tension (tenderness along course of round ligament [usually left] due to traction on structure in late pregnancy resulting from rotation of uterus and change of client's posture): Local heat and treatment as for pressure.

Ankle swelling (if not due to preeclampsia or eclampsia): Often due to sodium and water retention. Elevate legs frequently during day. Avoid tight clothing (e.g., garter, belts). Restrict salt intake. Wear support stockings.

Backache: Especially prominent during later part of pregnancy. Use massage, application of heat, specific exercises, medium-high heels, firm mattress.

Breast soreness: Is usually a problem during early and late pregnancy. Wear well-supporting bra. Ice packs to breasts.

Constipation: Stress good bowel habits, establish regular time for evacuation. Include bulk foods (e.g., bran), laxative foods, and liberal fluid intake. Encourage moderate exercise. May need stool softeners or mild laxative.

Flatulence, distention, and bowel cramping: Correct and simplify diet, reduce food intake at each meal. Maintain regular bowel function, regular exercise, and frequent change of position. Mild laxative prn.

Treatment/
Teaching
continued

Heartburn: Common in late pregnancy due to displacement of stomach and duodenum by the uterine fundus. Suggest calcium carbonate antacids (e.g., Tums). Sleep with several pillows under head or bed elevated on blocks. Frequent small meals. Hard candy, hot tea, and change of position also helpful.

Hemorrhoids: Avoid straining at stool by preventing and treating constipation. Warm sitz baths. Hemorrhoidal suppositories, creams, and/or Tucks per Rx.

Leg cramps: Occur often after sleep or recumbency after 1st trimester. Stand barefooted on a cold surface (e.g., tiled bathroom floor). Massage and "knead" the contracted muscle. Passively flex foot to lengthen calf muscle. Apply local heat.

Nausea: Common early in the morning when stomach is empty. Take small, frequent meals (dry popcorn, dry toast, and soda crackers in small amounts). Try alternating fluids and solids hourly. If nausea is present during or after meals, eat grapefruit slices or take sips of lemonade before eating rest of meal. Avoid hot, spicy foods. If vomiting occurs after every meal, contact MD.

Syncope and dizziness: Common in early pregnancy. Avoid inactivity, utilize deep breathing, vigorous leg motions, slow change of position. May be related to hypoglycemia; if so, encourage 6 small meals during the day instead of 3 large ones.

Urinary symptoms: Common, especially in advanced pregnancy due to reduced bladder capacity. R/o infection. If frequency, urgency, stress incontinence is acute, avoid tea, coffee, spices, and alcoholic beverages.

Uterine contractions (Braxton-Hicks): Commonly felt in late pregnancy, irregular and brief. Generally relieved by change of position.

Refer to MD

For symptoms not relieved with home treatment, development of serious complications; if contractions are regular and/or strong and not relieved with position change

Emergency

Eclampsia symptoms, vaginal hemorrhage

Cross
Reference

Back Pain, Calf Pain, Constipation, Edema, Fainting, Heartburn, Hemorrhoids, Morning Sickness, Nocturia, Preeclampsia, Urinary Tract Infection

Symptoms of pregnancy

Etiology

Assessment

All presumptive and probable signs of pregnancy can be due to other conditions. Clinical experience and passage of time are required to establish correct diagnosis. Identify date of LMP; was it normal? Is client using contraception? If so, identify. Presumptive signs of pregnancy: amenorrhea, nausea and vomiting (1st trimester), breast tenderness and tingling (after 1 to 2 weeks), urinary frequency and urgency (1st trimester), "quickening" (may appear at about 16th week), weight gain.

Treatment/ Teaching

Pregnancy can be confirmed easily by a blood or urine test shortly after the 1st period is missed. Medications (unless approved by MD) and x-rays should be restricted until diagnosis of pregnancy is made.

Refer to MD

For diagnosis and prenatal care, abortion counseling, handling of complications of pregnancy

Emergency

Vaginal hemorrhage, rupture of ectopic pregnancy

Cross Reference

Abortion; Amenorrhea; Ectopic Pregnancy; Menstrual Problems, Irregular Periods; Morning Sickness; Pregnancy Test; Vaginal Hemorrhage

Urine or blood test to detect pregnancy

Etiology

Assessment

**Treatment/
Teaching**

Urine test valid 2 weeks after missed period or 6 weeks (42 days) after 1st day of last menstrual period. Use 1st morning's voided specimen (otherwise may get false negative). Collect in clean container. Blood test (HCG) can be valid approximately 10 days after conception (30 to 35 days after 1st day of last menstrual period).

Refer to MD

For testing and to obtain test results (usually takes 24 hours to learn results)

Emergency

**Cross
Reference**

Pregnancy, Diagnosis Of

PREMATURE VENTRICULAR CONTRACTIONS (PVCs)

Contractions that occur when an irritable focus in the ventricle discharges before the next expected regular beat from the atrium

Etiology
3 to 5 PVCs/minute are frequently found in normal hearts. Frequent PVCs can be found in inflammatory or degenerative myocardial disease, cardiac failure from any cause, anxiety, fatigue, disturbed psychologic states, sympathomimetics, digitalis, tobacco, caffeine (in tea or coffee), hypokalemia, and hypoxia; also associated with disturbances in the CNS, GI, and GU systems.

Assessment
Client may complain of "feeling something turn over" in chest, a "shock in the chest," a skipped beat, or a choking sensation.

Treatment/ Teaching
If client is young with no previous cardiac history, chest pain, or dyspnea, reassure that this can be normal. Avoid stimulants (e.g., coffee, tea, cocoa, etc.).

Refer to MD
If PVCs persist and cause discomfort (without previous cardiac history)

Emergency
History of angina and numerous "thuds" in the pulse (thud indicates stronger beat after PVC)

Cross Reference
Dysrhythmias, Palpitations, Paroxysmal Atrial Tachycardia

Symptom complex that may appear a few days prior to monthly menses

Etiology May be an exaggerated physiologic and psychologic reaction to menstruation

Assessment R/o hyperthyroidism, hyperinsulinism, extreme psychoneurosis, and psychosis. Usual symptoms include anxiety, edema and/or weight gain, agitation, insomnia, inability to concentrate, feeling of inadequacy, breast pain, nausea and vomiting, diarrhea or constipation, depression, self-pity, or irritability; food cravings are commonplace.

Treatment/ Teaching Avoid extra stress during this time. Extra rest. Reassurance, positive suggestions. Diuretics and/or tranquilizers if indicated. Low sodium diet.

Refer to MD For management of incapacitating problem

Emergency

Cross Reference Dysmenorrhea

Guidelines for evaluating postoperative care of client with transurethral resection

Etiology

Assessment

**Treatment/
Teaching**   Client usually stays in hospital 5 to 7 days. If client has bleeding at beginning or end of stream
or if urine is dark, okay to stay home. Have client rest and drink increased fluids.

Refer to MD   If still bleeding after rest and pushing fluids

Emergency   Constant bright red bleeding and clots in urine

**Cross
Reference**   Blood in Urine; Urine, Dark-Colored

Inflammation of the prostate gland

Etiology Bacteria, nonbacteria

Assessment **Acute:** Usual symptoms are dysuria and frequency, which may be followed by fever. Client may complain of a discharge, postvoid dribbling, hematuria at end of the stream. There may be a history of gonorrhea, abrupt change in sex habits, heavy caffeine or alcohol ingestion, and nonspecific stress prior to onset of symptoms.

Chronic: May follow an acute prostatic infection or may develop insidiously, producing symptoms of minor urinary irritation, including frequency, nocturia, and dysuria. Check for trouble starting stream, retention, nocturia, UTI symptoms, dysuria.

**Treatment/
Teaching** **Acute:** Bedrest, fluids, antibiotic therapy.

Chronic: Fluids, hot sitz baths, antibiotic therapy.

Refer to MD For evaluation and treatment

Emergency Severe pain or retention

**Cross
Reference** Blood in Urine; Incontinence; Nocturia; Urinary Tract Infection; Urine, Decreased Output or Stream; Voiding Difficulty

Impaired mental functioning that markedly interferes with the ability to carry out daily activities

Etiology

Psychiatric cause unknown; toxic agents, situational stress

Assessment

Psychosis involves the total personality; it prevents or seriously interferes with the client's relationships with other persons and groups. The psychoses include 1) major affective disorders; 2) schizophrenia; 3) paranoid states; 4) other psychoses (e.g., psychotic-depressive reactions, organic brain syndromes). Symptoms vary, but include 1) severe disorder of mood (depression-elation); 2) thinking disturbances (delusions and affect disturbances); or 3) paranoid ideation. Questions to ask in assessing if an individual is experiencing a psychotic episode include 1) "Are your thoughts 'speeded up' (going so fast you can't keep up with them)?" 2) "Have you ever seen or heard anything you think might not be there or that others don't see or hear?" 3) "Have you ever had strange, frightening thoughts or experiences?" 4) "Have you ever felt as if people were after you or out to get you?" Persons experiencing a psychosis are apt to answer "yes" to one or more of these questions. You may want to talk with family member or someone else who has been with the client to ask: 1) What is the person's eating and sleeping patterns? 2) Has this ever happened to the client before? 3) Is there a history of mental illness? Is the client taking any drugs? 4) Is the client currently under treatment?

Treatment/ Teaching

Maintain a calm, supportive environment until client can be seen.

Refer to MD

For evaluation and treatment; refer to a mental health resource in the community:

Emergency

Call police if client is threatening bodily harm to self or to others; for situations involving weapons

Cross Reference

Anxiety, Confusion, Delirium, Hallucinations, Suicide

A condition, usually acute but sometimes subacute or chronic, marked by an excess of fluid in the extravascular spaces of the lungs.

Etiology   Cardiac disease, pneumonia, hypertension, emphysema, fluid overload, sodium retention

Assessment   History of cardiac or respiratory disease; presenting symptoms include tachypnea, cough, frothy (pink) sputum, wheezing, dyspnea, pallor or cyanosis, sense of oppression in chest. Onset may be acute or insidious.

Treatment/ Teaching   **For mild and/or chronic problem:** Rest, semi-Fowler's position, or sit in chair. O_2 if ordered and available.

Refer to MD   For management of chronic problem, to evaluate need for hospitalization, or if no relief with medications and/or O_2 at home

Emergency   For severe dyspnea with or without cardiac symptoms; acute onset

Cross Reference   Breathing Difficulty, Chest Pain, Congestive Heart Failure, Emphysema, Oxygen Information, Pneumonia, Pulmonary Embolus

A blood clot that lodges in a pulmonary artery

Etiology Usually originates from thrombosis of the deep veins in the legs; fragments of thrombus are carried to pulmonary artery. Common in elderly, bedridden clients, early postpartum, or postoperative clients. Predisposing factors include bed rest, heart disease, chronic obstructive lung disease, hip fracture, malignancy, aging, acute paralysis, and hematologic disorders

Assessment Sudden dyspnea and anxiety with or without substernal pain, history of thrombophlebitis, cough, hemoptysis. R/o MI, pneumonia, atelectasis, pneumothroax, and other cardiac and pulmonary causes of dyspnea and chest pain (may complain of mild or transient dyspnea and pleural pain with small embolism).

Treatment/ Teaching Position of comfort, O_2 if available. Arrange emergency transportation with O_2.

Refer to MD If symptoms mild and transient

Emergency Severe dyspnea and chest pain

Cross Reference Breathing Difficulty, Chest Pain, Cyanosis, Pleurisy, Pneumothorax

Etiology

Assessment

Treatment/ Teaching

Refer to MD

Emergency

Cross Reference Asthma, Atelectasis, Breathing Difficulty, Bronchitis, Chest Pain, Cyanosis, Emphysema, Oxygen Information, Pleurisy, Pneumonia, Pneumothorax, Pulmonary Edema, Pulmonary Embolus

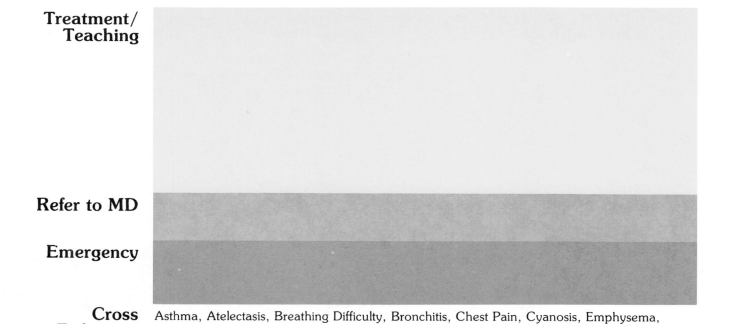

Acute viral disease of the central nervous system that can affect all mammals and is transmitted from one to another by infected secretion, usually saliva

Etiology   Rabies virus; humans contact it when bitten by a rabid animal, commonly wild animals or household pets infected by a bite from a wild animal. Bats, skunks, and foxes are extensively infected. Rodents are unlikely to have rabies.

Assessment   Prodromal period of 1 to 4 days marked by fever, headache, malaise, nausea, vomiting, cough. Encephalitic phase is marked by excessive motor activity, excitation, agitation; brainstem dysfunction follows shortly thereafter. R/o viral encephalitis. History of bite is usually highly suggestive of diagnosis.

Treatment/   Wash any animal bite well with soap and water. Capture the involved animal, confine, and
Teaching   observe for 7 to 10 days. Animal to be evaluated by a veterinarian prn unusual behavior. (A captured wild animal should be killed and the head shipped on ice to nearest qualified laboratory for examination.) When animal cannot be examined, presume skunks, bats, coyotes, foxes, and raccoons to be rabid. Evaluate the rabies potential of bites by other animals individually. Human diploid-cell culture rabies vaccine, 6 immunizations (1cc each) on days 0, 3 , 7, 14, 30, 90 (World Health Organization recommendation).

Refer to MD   For evaluation and treatment

Emergency   Evidence of CNS dysfunction

Cross   Bites, Animal and Human (Peds)
Reference

Skin eruption

Etiology Communicable disease, contact with chemicals or irritants, medications, allergens, unknown causes

Assessment See individual cross reference cards.

**Treatment/
Teaching**

Refer to MD

Emergency

**Cross
Reference** Acne, Allergies, Athlete's Foot, Chickenpox, Dermatitis, Eczema, Heat Rash, Herpes, Hives, Itching, Jock Itch, Measles (Peds), Meningitis, Mononucleosis, Nettles Contact, Poison Oak or Ivy, Roseola (Peds), Rubella, Scabies, Scarlet Fever or Scarlatina, Toxic Shock Syndrome

Bloody discharge from rectum

Etiology Hemorrhoids, rectal fissure, malignancy, constipation, GI bleeding (e.g., ulcers, colitis), recent viral illness with diarrhea

Assessment Rely on history and ancillary symptoms. Determine the amount of blood loss and if bright red or dark in color. Determine if acute or chronic problem. If less than 1 tsp of bright red blood, suspect hemorrhoids or rectal fissure.

Treatment/ Teaching Sitz bath, hot water bottle to rectal area prn pain (do not use heating pad—it can burn this area).

Refer to MD If problem chronic, if blood loss is minimal; for diagnosis

Emergency Hemorrhage, intractable pain

Cross Reference Black Stools, Blood in Stools, Colitis, Constipation, Diarrhea, Hemorrhoids

Etiology

Assessment

**Treatment/
Teaching**

Refer to MD

Emergency

**Cross
Reference**   Hemorrhoids, Pinworms (Peds)

Blood treatment or peritoneal lavage to remove body wastes in clients with renal failure

Etiology   Renal dysfunction or failure

Assessment

**Treatment/
Teaching**

Refer to closest kidney center:

Telephone Number:
(They are source for advice and help if the client's own physician is not available.)

Refer to MD   Whenever possible for advice and management

Emergency   Renal failure, hemorrhage from shunt or fistula

**Cross
Reference**

RHO GAM GUIDELINES
(For Rh Incompatibility Prophylaxis)

Directions for administration of Rho Gam/Micro Gam for Rh negative mothers with Rh positive babies

Etiology   Rh incompatibility

Assessment

Treatment/ Teaching   Rho Gam/Micro Gam must be given within 72 hours post-delivery or abortion when there is Rh incompatibility. Spontaneous abortion with Rh negative mother: greater than 8 weeks gestation, Rho Gam used; less than 8 weeks: Micro Gam can be used. Rho Gam may require matching for compatibility while Micro Gam may not.

Refer to MD   For blood work, if necessary, and administration of Rho Gam/Micro Gam

Emergency

Cross Reference   Abortion

Method for removing ring from a swollen finger

Etiology

Assessment

Treatment/ Teaching
Take a length of fine string or thread, insert one end under the ring on palmar side, then wrap the other long end snugly around the finger on distal side of ring. Next, take the short end of the string (palmar side) and gradually unwind it. This will force the ring to inch down the finger. Repeat until the ring passes the proximal joint. May also try soaping the finger and sliding the ring over the joint.

Refer to MD
If unable to remove ring with above methods

Emergency
Impaired circulation to finger

Cross Reference

An infection of the skin, hair, or nails

Etiology   Fungal infection with trichophyton

Assessment   Itching distinguishes ringworm from psoriasis, erythema multiforme, and pityriasis rosea. Lesion is pruritic, ringed, scaling, may have small vesicles in outer border. Lesions occur on exposed skin surfaces; may have history of handling young kittens or other infected domestic animals.

Treatment/ Teaching   Avoid contact with infected household pets. No exchange of clothing without adequate laundering. Antifungal ointment (e.g., Tinactin, clortrimazole [Lotrimin or Mycelex]) twice a day. Not especially contagious.

Refer to MD   If no improvement after using antifungal agent for 3 days

Emergency

Cross Reference   Fungal Infections

An exanthematous, contagious disease with usually mild constitutional symptoms

Etiology   Rubella virus

Assessment   Incubation period is from 14 to 21 days (usually 16 to 18). Contagious period is from 7 days before to approximately 5 days after the appearance of the rash. The rash begins on the face and neck, quickly spreading to the trunk and extremities. Minimal or no prodromal symptoms (e.g., fever, malaise, headache, stiff joints, mild pharyngeal catarrah), no Koplik's spots, rapid spread of the rash, and its usual disappearance by the 3rd day all help to distinguish rubella from rubeola.

Treatment/ Teaching   Fluids. Acetaminophen prn fever preferred for clients under 16 years of age. Calamine lotion, cool baths prn itching. Avoid contact with articles freshly contaminated with nasopharyngeal secretions, feces, or urine of infected person. Rest. Notify any pregnant contacts, especially those in their 1st trimester. Rubella may result in abortion, stillborns, or congenital defects in infants born to mothers who were infected during the early months of pregnancy.

Refer to MD   For diagnosis; for gamma globulin for exposed female in 1st trimester of pregnancy

Emergency

Cross Reference   Antipyretics, Aspirin and Acetaminophen (Peds), Gamma Globulin Information, Immunization Information (Adult and Peds), Rash

Acute gastroenteritis

Etiology Ingestion of food or liquid contaminated with salmonella organism

Assessment Symptoms include fever, nausea and vomiting, cramping, abdominal pain and diarrhea (may be bloody). Symptoms appear 8 to 48 hours after ingestion of contaminated food and usually persist over 3 to 5 days. Salmonella can be cultured from the stools. The disease is usually self-limiting and treatment is symptomatic.

Treatment/ Teaching See cross reference cards for diarrhea, nausea and vomiting, and fever.

Refer to MD For evaluation, moderate dehydration, and for stool culture (especially if stool bloody and/or recent contact with person known to have salmonella)

Emergency Grossly bloody stool, severe pain, or dehydration

Cross Reference Abdominal Pain, Blood in Stools, Dehydration, Diarrhea, Fever, Gastroenteritis, Nausea and Vomiting

A parasitic skin disease

Etiology   Infestation with Sarcoptes scabei

Assessment   Tiny pruritic blisters and pustules in "runs" or "tracks" especially on sides of fingers, wrists, finger webs, heels, elbows, waist, armpits, buttocks crease, inner thigh. Itching may occur during the day, but is usually more severe and intense at night. The runs or tracks appear as short, irregular marks as if made by a sharp pencil. History of close contact with infected individual is helpful in diagnosis. Lesions usually do not appear on face. Scabies is an infestation of the entire body in children 2 years of age or younger; occurs only from the neck down in children older than 2.

Treatment/ Teaching   Client needs to be seen for diagnosis to be made. Treat with appropriate medicine; see Antiparasitics in Pediatric Doses of Commonly Used Medications. Warm, soapy bath should precede application of meds. Apply evenly from the neck down and rub in gently. Pay particular attention to the fingers, wrists, feet, groin. Children under age 2 must have the medication applied to the face, head, and neck area. The medication is a poison, so put socks on children's hands to keep fingers out of the mouth. Change sheets, night clothes, and underclothes. Wash linen and underclothes thoroughly. Repeat treatment 7 days later. Treat all members of the family. Oral antihistamine (e.g., Benadryl) prn pruritis. Dress cool, sleep cool, bathe cool. Prolonged itching could mean reinfection or allergic reaction to dead mites.Kwell (shampoo and lotion) is the drug of choice for treatment of scabies. This drug may have systemic side effects. RID and A-200 Pyrinate are equally effective against scabies and can be safely used by all individuals except those suffering from ragweed allergy (hay fever). Eurax can be used on children under 5 years of age.

Refer to MD   For diagnosis and treatment, for any questions re using Kwell; i.e., debilitated, elderly, or newborn.

Emergency

Cross Reference   Dermatitis, Contact; Lice; Pediatric Doses of Commonly Used Medications (Antiparasitics)

An acute, contagious disease characterized by sore throat, strawberry tongue, fever, punctiform scarlet rash, circumoral pallor.

Etiology

Beta hemolytic strep, almost always Group A

Assessment

Usual incubation period is 3 to 5 days. Transmitted by direct contact and large droplet infection; may accompany or follow a strep pharyngitis. Usual symptoms include a diffuse fine rash on trunk and chest (less on back and arms) that feels like sandpaper; swollen and painful anterior cervical nodes; inflamed tonsils, very red cheeks, circumoral pallor, strawberry tongue, fever.

Treatment/ Teaching

Fluids (especially cold fluids, popsicles). ASA prn fever and sore throat, saline gargles. Antibiotic per Rx. Contagious until 24 hours of antibiotic therapy completed. Ice collar prn discomfort of swollen lymph nodes.

Refer to MD

For diagnosis and treatment, immediately if fever high and considerable discomfort; for treatment of secondary problem (e.g., rheumatic fever, glomerulonephritis)

Emergency

Cross Reference

Aspirin and Acetaminophen (Peds), Fever, Ice Collar (Glossary), Pediatric Doses of Commonly Used Medications, Rash, Saline Gargle (Glossary), Sore Throat, Strep Throat (Peds)

Etiology

Assessment

**Treatment/
Teaching**

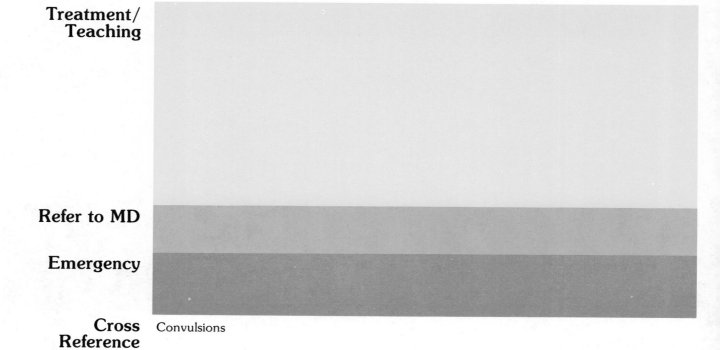

Refer to MD

Emergency

**Cross
Reference**   Convulsions

Guidelines for resumption of sexual intercourse after delivery or surgical procedure

Etiology

Assessment

Treatment/ Teaching

Before delivery: No sexual activity during last month of pregnancy, if any bleeding or pain.

After delivery: Usually not until after postpartum check.

After D&C or abortion: No intercourse for 2 weeks after procedure.

After laproscopic tubal ligation: No restrictions.

Refer to MD

If bleeding occurs after intercourse following any of the above procedures, if infection develops

Emergency

Vaginal hemorrhage

Cross Reference

Bleeding, Vaginal, During Pregnancy; Vaginal Hemorrhage

An involuntary shivering or trembling of the muscles

Etiology   Fever, drugs, virus, chronic illness (e.g., parkinsonism), cerebral palsy, multiple sclerosis, recent discontinuance of high alcohol or coffee intake, hyper- or hypothyroidism, overuse of muscles, anxiety, emotional upset

Assessment   Rely on history and ancillary symptoms.

Treatment/ Teaching   Chills usually precede fever and increase as fever increases, subside when the fever "breaks." Antipyretics prn fever. If shakiness results from overuse of muscles, apply moist heat.

Refer to MD   If sudden onset; prolonged symptoms; for evaluation and treatment of chronic problem

Emergency

Cross Reference   Antipyretic Drugs, Anxiety, Fever, Hyperthyroidism, Hypothyroidism

Acute infection of the nervous system characterized by vesicular lesions along the distribution of a nerve root.

Etiology Herpes virus

Assessment Prodromal symptoms (chills, fever, malaise, GI disturbances) may be present 3 to 4 days before onset of vesicular lesions. Pain may precede the appearance of the lesions. Eruptions most often occur in the thoracic region and spread unilaterally. Diagnosis readily apparent after vesicles appear in characteristic distribution. R/o tic douloureux, chickenpox.

Treatment/ Teaching Calamine lotion to lesions prn pain or itching. Analgesics (usually codeine if client not allergic to it). Benadryl prn pruritis. Light, loose, cotton clothing. May require prednisone to subdue reaction. Some clients have long-lasting, very painful posttherapeutic neuralgia. Avoid touching lesions, use careful handwashing technique.

Refer to MD For diagnosis and treatment; to ophthalmologist if eye is affected

Emergency

Cross Reference Chickenpox (Peds); Facial Pain; Herpes, Genital; Herpes Simplex; Numbness; Tic Douloureux

A state in which blood flow to peripheral tissues is inadequate to sustain life because of insufficient cardiac output or maldistribution of peripheral blood flow, usually associated with progressive arterial hypotension

Etiology   Severe trauma, major surgery, massive hemorrhage, dehydration, myocardial infarction, overwhelming infections, poisoning, drug reactions

Assessment   Symptoms usually include altered sensorium, ashen pallor, clammy skin, rapid and weak pulse, air hunger, thirst, scanty urine output, and a tendency to steadily progress to an "irreversible" phase.

Treatment/ Teaching   Place client in flat position with slight elevation of legs **if no dyspnea present**. Clear airway. CPR if necessary. Keep client comfortable and warm. Avoid chilling or excessive externally applied heat. No oral fluids even though client complains of thirst (intestinal absorption is decreased). Arrange for emergency aid.

Refer to MD

Emergency   Emergency transportation to hospital

Cross Reference   Abruptio Placentae; Allergic Reaction; Aneurysm; Bleeding from Esophageal Varices; Blood in Stools; Blood in Vomitus; Burns; Coma; Ectopic Pregnancy; Electric Shock; Fainting; Food Poisoning; Menorrhagia; Myocardial Infarction; Pneumonia

Etiology

Assessment

**Treatment/
Teaching**

Refer to MD

Emergency

**Cross
Reference** Allergic Reaction, Asthma, Atelectasis, Breathing Difficulty, Bronchitis, Chest Pain, Choking, Congestive Heart Failure, Emphysema, Myocardial Infarction, Pleurisy, Pneumonia, Pneumothorax, Pulmonary Edema, Pulmonary Embolus

Pressure and discomfort in facial sinus area

Etiology URI, sinus infection, chronic sinusitis, allergies

Assessment Rely on history and ancillary symptoms.

Treatment/ Teaching Steam inhalation with head in a downward position (hold towel-covered head over basin of steamy water). Hot pack to sinus area. Decongestant (e.g., Sudafed, Chlortrimeton, Coriciden D). Saline, Neo-Synephrine, or Afrin nose drops (use no longer than 5 days). Clear fluids; avoid dairy products. Analgesics (ASA or acetaminophen) prn.

Refer to MD For evaluation and treatment of acute infection (i.e., if client has facial swelling, pain, fever, purulent yellow or green discharge from nose), or for management of chronic problem

Emergency

Cross Reference Allergies, Cold Symptoms, Hot Pack (Glossary), Nasal Congestion, Saline Nose Drops (Glossary), Sinus Infection, Upper Respiratory Infection

Inflammation of a sinus

Etiology   Usually follows an acute URI, swimming or diving, dental abscess or extractions, nasal allergies, or occurs as an exacerbation of chronic sinus infection.

Assessment   Symptoms include headache (typically worse during day and subsides in evening), facial pain, tenderness and swelling with nasal obstruction, and purulent nasal and postnasal discharge, sometimes causing cough and sore throat. **Acute maxillary sinusitis** may cause pain in teeth. **Acute ethmoiditis** causes headache between and behind eyes, eye motion increases pain. **Frontal sinusitis** creates tenderness medially in roof of orbit. **Acute dental infection** usually produces greater facial swelling lower in the face, with marked tenderness of involved tooth. **Tear sac infection** is distinguished from ethmoiditis by more localized swelling and tenderness, greater involvement of eyelids, and absence of nasal discharge.

Treatment/ Teaching   Steam inhalation with head in downward position to promote drainage (hang towel-covered head over basin of steamy water). Hot packs to sinus area. Decongestant (e.g., Sudafed, Chlortrimeton, Coriciden D). Neo-Synephrine or Afrin nose drops (use no longer than 5 days). Clear fluids; avoid dairy products. Analgesics (ASA or acetaminophen) prn. Warm saline sniffs (¼ tsp salt in 8 oz warm water in a basin): using hand to dip solution, sniff into and out of the nose in short in-and-out motions.

Refer to MD   For evaluation and treatment of acute infection

Emergency   Fever, swelling and tenderness above and medial to the eye

Cross Reference   Cold Symptoms, Facial Pain, Hot Packs (Glossary), Influenza, Nasal Congestion, Upper Respiratory Infection

Inflammation of pharynx

Etiology   Viral or bacterial infection, irritation, post-op pain

Assessment   Rely on history and ancillary symptoms. Determine if any family member is being treated for strep throat.

Treatment/ Teaching   ASA every 4 hours prn discomfort, fever (acetaminophen if viral etiology is suspected). Saline gargles; cold fluids (ice chips, popsicles, iced drinks). Vaporizer, or hold towel-covered head over sink of hot water; ice collar. Throat lozenges; topical anesthetic throat sprays (not on new postoperative site). Discontinue smoking. If strep throat, client is considered contagious until s/he has had 24 hours of antibiotic therapy.

Refer to MD   If sore throat and/or fever persists longer than 48 hours or for diagnosis and treatment of strep throat

Emergency

Cross Reference   Antipyretic Drugs; Cold Symptoms; Diphtheria; Drooling; Fever; Herpes Simplex; Hoarseness; Mononucleosis; Pediatric Doses of Commonly Used Medications; Scarlet Fever or Scarlatina; Strep Throat (Peds); Swallowing Difficulty; Swollen Glands; Tonsillectomy and Adenoidectomy; Upper Respiratory Infection

Guidelines for treatment

Etiology

Assessment **Black widow:** Local symptoms include sharp, pinprick sensation followed by dull numbing pain, slight swelling. Systemic effects include muscle rigidity, paralysis, abdominal pain, seizures, stupor.

Brown recluse: Local symptoms do not develop until 2 to 8 hours after bite, then area becomes red and proceeds to tissue necrosis. Systemic effects include fever, malaise, nausea, petechial rash.

Treatment/ Teaching **Black widow:** Ice packs to site. Warm bath and muscle relaxants for muscle spasms; may need narcotic analgesic.

Brown recluse: Immobilize bitten part; avoid manipulation of area (may require excision of necrotic area at medical facility).

Refer to MD For initial evaluation

Emergency CNS symptoms, tissue necrosis, and/or petechiae

Cross Reference Petechiae

Minimal Vaginal Bleeding

Etiology   "Ovulation bleeding," "break-through" associated with birth control pills, IUD, endometritis, hormonal disturbances, threatened abortion, ectopic pregnancy, intrauterine pathology (e.g., polyps, fibroids, hyperplasia, carcinoma), menopause

Assessment   Rely on history and ancillary symptoms.

Treatment/
Teaching
Ovulation bleeding: Occurs at time of ovulation, is very light and lasts for no more than 2 days. Usually occurs about 14 days before onset of next period.

Threatened AB: Bedrest with bathroom privileges. Be seen in ER prn heavy bleeding, clotting, fever, pain.

Break-through bleeding: See cross reference cards.

IUD: Commonly has some spotting but may be sign of initial perforation of uterus.

Refer to MD   For diagnosis and treatment

Emergency   Vaginal hemorrhage or severe pain

Cross
Reference   Abortion, Break-Through Bleeding, Ectopic Pregnancy, Menopausal Symptoms

Trauma to a joint that causes pain and disability depending upon degree of injury to the ligaments

Etiology Trauma, "twisting" ankle

Assessment **First degree** sprain is characterized by some fiber tear but no functional loss or decreased strength. There is mild point tenderness, no abnormal motion, minimal swelling.

Second degree sprain presents partial tear with some function loss, point tenderness, light to moderate abnormal motion, localized hemorrhage.

Third degree sprain indicates complete tear with total function loss, marked abnormal motion, possible deformity.

Treatment/ Teaching **For mild sprain:** Elevate extremity. Ice pack intermittently for 48 to 72 hours, then heat to area. Mild analgesics (ASA) prn discomfort. Limitation of activity until healing occurs.

Refer to MD For evaluation of second and third degree sprain or possible fracture

Emergency

Cross Reference Ice Pack (Glossary)

Etiology

Assessment

**Treatment/
Teaching**

Refer to MD

Emergency

**Cross
Reference**   Abdominal Pain (Adult & Peds)

Bowel movements lacking the usual brown coloration; clay-colored stools

Etiology Hepatitis, heavy use of antacids, recent severe diarrhea

Assessment Rely on history and ancillary symptoms

Treatment/ Teaching When due to use of antacids or recent severe diarrhea, normal coloration will usually return without medical intervention when ingestion of antacids is decreased or physiology returns to normal.

Refer to MD For diagnosis and evaluation if cause unknown

Emergency

Cross Reference Hepatitis

Damage to musculotendinous structures either by overuse (chronic strain) or overstress (acute strain)

Etiology Excessive use or overstretch of tissues

Assessment **First degree** strain results in no appreciable reduction in strength. The client experiences local pain and tenderness that increases with movement. Mild spasm and swelling may be present.

Second degree strain results in partial decrease in strength, local pain, moderate spasm, swelling, ecchymosis.

Third degree strain results in severe pain, swelling, hematoma, loss of muscle function.

Treatment/ Teaching **For mild strain:** Rest and/or immobilization of area. Ice pack prn spasm and swelling. Analgesic (ASA) prn.

Refer to MD For evaluation of second and third degree strains

Emergency

Cross Reference Back Pain, Calf Pain, Cramps, Ice Pack (Glossary), Muscle Pain or Spasm, Neck Pain, Sprain

Destruction of brain substance resulting from intracerebral hemorrhage, thrombosis, embolism, or vascular insufficiency

Etiology Arteriosclerotic vascular disease, hypertension, embolus, ruptured cerebral aneurysm

Assessment Onset usually abrupt, evolution rapid, and symptoms reach a peak within seconds, minutes, or hours. Uncommon in persons under 40. Usual symptoms include sudden neurologic complaints varying from focal-motor deficits, hypesthesia, speech defects to coma. May be associated with vomiting, convulsions, or headaches.

Treatment/ Teaching **In recovery phase:** Encourage self-care as much as possible. Range-of-motion and other exercises. Prevention of decubitus ulcers. Visiting Nurses Association (VNA) referral for speech therapy, vocational rehabilitation, physical therapy.

Refer to MD For evaluation, if symptoms are not grossly incapacitating

Emergency Sudden onset of symptoms, comatose, or grossly incapacitated at onset of symptoms

Cross Reference Aphasia, Balance Problems, Coma, Confusion, Headache, Incontinence, Irritability, Muscle Weakness, Nausea and Vomiting, Numbness, Paralysis

Abscess in the follicles of an eyelash

Etiology   Staphylococcus

Assessment   Inflamation characterized by localized red, swollen, acutely tender area on the upper or lower lid. Chief symptom is pain of an intensity directly related to the amount of swelling.

Treatment/   Hot pack to area for 20 minutes, 4 to 6 times a day.
Teaching

Refer to MD   If sty does not spontaneously open, drain, and heal; if resolution has not begun within 48 hours of hot packs

Emergency

Cross
Reference

An act or instance of taking one's own life voluntarily and intentionally. The attempt may range from an impulsive gesture to a premeditated and carefully designed try at self-destruction.

Etiology Depression, psychotic illness, feeling overwhelmed by problems in living, an attempt to control others, alcohol or drug abuse, serious or terminal illness

Assessment The seriousness of the underlying psychologic disorder is often difficult to determine. The key to suicide prevention is alertness to the two clinical conditions most likely to end in suicide: depression and alcoholism. Evaluation of suicide risk includes the following questions:

1. Is there a history of previous suicide attempts? If so, what was the method? Was medical treatment required?
2. Does the client have a specific plan? How lethal and available is the method: gun? poisoning? hanging?
3. Is there a history of depression? Is person currently depressed?
4. Is there a family history of suicide?
5. Is there severe agitation, distortions in reality, impairment of impulse control and judgment, or frustration of dependency needs?
6. Has there been a recent loss through death of a close person?
7. Is there a problem with alcohol or drug abuse?
8. Does the client live alone? Does s/he have an established support system?
9. Was client recently placed on antidepressants (may give client enough energy to act)?
10. Does the client have a chronic, debilitating illness?

Treatment/ Teaching If the client answers yes to several of the above questions, especially #2, the suicide potential is high. The ability to communicate understanding and obtain help for the person is the essence of handling the potential suicide. If the client refuses to talk further and is a high suicide risk (has a plan, weapon, etc.), the police should be notified. Listen for background noises, request identifying information, etc; trace the call if possible. Maintain phone contact with client. Bring client to ER facility; try to locate friend or relative to stay with client.

Give caller phone number of local Suicide Prevention Center and Hot Line:

Refer to MD Contact client's own therapist if currently in treatment, or have client brought to ER; client needs immediate emotional support and guidance.

Emergency If suicide attempt has already been made, arrange emergency transportation to hospital.

Cross Reference Depression, Psychosis

Injury to the skin with erythema, tenderness, and blistering

Etiology   Excessive exposure to sun or other source of ultraviolet light

Assessment   **First degree:** redness of skin (erythema)

Second degree: blistering of skin; fever, GI symptoms, malaise, or prostration

**Treatment/
Teaching**   Cool water compresses. Milk of Magnesia applied to nonblistered skin is soothing. In drying stage, use moisturizing cream (Nivea, Keri, Vaseline Intensive Care Lotion). For eyes: cold compresses, eye patch, or be in dark room. ASA prn. Prevent sunburn with limited initial exposure to sunlight (30 minutes midday) in summer and use of sunscreens containing PABA, benzophenes (e.g., Pre-Sun, Sunguard, Pabafilm), or zinc oxide (complete block). All sun products are now labeled 2 through 15. 2 provides least protection; 15 is almost a complete block.

Refer to MD   For eye pain, large number of blisters, or edema

Emergency   Symptoms of heat stroke

**Cross
Reference**   Burns, Heat Stroke

Sensation of pain or tightness in throat when swallowing

Etiology Croup, epiglottitis, foreign body, allergic reaction, severe sore throat

Assessment Determine degree of respiratory distress (if any), drooling, client's color, recent health history, exposure to allergens, apparent level of discomfort or illness, presence or absence of facial edema.

Treatment/ Teaching ASA every 4 hours prn sore throat (without respiratory distress). Ice chips, popsicles, cold fluids. Ice collar. Topical anesthetic throat lozenge or spray. Saline gargle.

Refer to MD For undiagnosed sore throat without respiratory distress

Emergency Respiratory distress

Cross Reference Allergic Reaction, Choking, Croup (Peds), Epiglottitis (Peds), Ice Collar (Glossary), Saline Gargle (Glossary), Sore Throat

Enlargement of lymph nodes

Etiology

Viral or bacterial infection (local or systemic), reaction to antigen or tumor

Assessment

Rely on history and ancillary symptoms. Try to discern source of infection. R/o local infection of the gland. R/o tumor. Duration of less than 1 week plus associated symptoms of infection (e.g., sore throat, fever) suggest infectious etiology. One or two swollen nodes of longer than 2 weeks with no infectious symptoms may indicate tumor.

Treatment/ Teaching

If secondary to URI, sore throat: Fluids; watch for increased swelling, redness, streaking, discharge, persistent fever; ice collar. Lymph nodes swell in normal response to bodily invasion by bacteria or viruses in the acute phase of the illness.

Refer to MD

If nodes become infected, if they become increasingly swollen, if tumor is a likely possibility, or for evaluation of systemic symptoms

Emergency

Cross Reference

Fever, Hyperthyroidism, Ice Collar (Glossary), Mononucleosis, Sore Throat, Strep Throat (Peds), Upper Respiratory Infection

An infectious, venereal disease characterized by primary, secondary, latent, and tertiary stages

Etiology   Spirochetal bacteria, Treponema pallidum; usually sexually transmitted

Assessment   Incubation period averages 3 weeks

Primary stage: Penile, anal, or oral chancre begins usually as a single, painless papule that becomes eroded. Regional, bilateral, painless lymphadenopathy also present. Chancre heals in 4 to 6 weeks, lymphadenopathy may persist for months.

Secondary stage: Numerous manifestations including macular, papular, papulosquamous and occasionally pustular rashes widely distributed. May occur on palms, soles, face, and scalp. May have wart-like lesions, condylomata in warm, moist intertriginous areas. Other symptoms include fever, weight loss, malaise, anorexia, headache.

Latent stage: An asymptomatic period, diagnosed by a positive blood test for syphilis, lasting from months to years.

Tertiary stage: Characterized by progressive, destructive, mucocutaneous, musculoskeletal or parenchymal lesions; aortic or CNS disease.

Treatment/ Teaching   Penicillin G is the drug of choice. A long period of exposure to penicillin is required for treatment because of the unusually slow rate of multiplication of the organism. Sexual intercourse should be avoided with any penile lesion. Secondary, latent, and tertiary stages are transmitted only through blood products.

Refer to MD   For definitive diagnosis and treatment

Emergency

Cross Reference   Herpes, Genital; Penile Lesion; Venereal Warts

Blockage of tear duct opening

Etiology   Unknown

Assessment   Usual symptom is chronic, runny, clear discharge from affected eye.

**Treatment/
Teaching**   Massage tear duct. Warm saline compresses.

Refer to MD   If discharge becomes purulent, if no relief of symptoms with home treatment.

Emergency

**Cross
Reference**

Lesion, injury, or infection in the testicles

Etiology   Infection, trauma, torsion, hernia, tumor

Assessment   Rely on history and ancillary symptoms.

**Treatment/
Teaching**   Elevate scrotum on rolled towel. Ice pack to area. Wear supporter.

Refer to MD   If sudden onset or increasing pain; any male under age 18 with onset of testicular pain should be seen immediately; for evaluation of any nodule

Emergency   Intense pain

**Cross
Reference**   Ice Pack (Glossary), Vasectomy

Etiology

Assessment

**Treatment/
Teaching**

Refer to MD

Emergency

**Cross
Reference**   Bites, Animal and Human (Peds); Immunization Information (Peds); Laceration; Tetanus Immunization (Peds)

Increased desire for fluids

Etiology   Diabetes, increased salt intake, some medications, hangover, hot weather, intestinal bypass surgery, Lithium-related polyuria

Assessment   Rely on history and ancillary symptoms

Treatment/ Teaching

If diabetic: Should be seen in ER; may be in ketoacidosis. Check for dehydration.

If not diabetic: Fluids. Decrease Na intake (unless related to heat prostration).

Refer to MD   For evaluation of persistent problem

Emergency   Advancing ketoacidosis

Cross Reference   Dehydration, Diabetic Ketoacidosis, Diabetes Mellitus, Heat Prostration

Inflammation of the wall of a vein with secondary thrombosis within the involved segment

Etiology   Most common causes are venous stasis and pressure changes in the vein wall that develop when legs lie for hours without moving (e.g., on bed or operating table). Predisposing factors are age, malignancy, shock, dehydration, anemia, obesity, chronic infection, birth control pills.

Assessment   Client may complain of dull ache, tight feeling, or pain in calf or whole leg, especially when walking. May feel anxious. Client may be asymptomatic until symptoms of pulmonary embolus appear. Calf muscle strain or contusion may be hard to differentiate from thrombophlebitis. With cellulitis (infection), a wound may be present and inflammation of skin is more marked. Bilateral leg edema is more likely to be the result of heart, kidney, or liver disease. Check for pain, swelling, tenderness, area warm to touch, positive Homans' sign (pain upon dorsiflexion of the foot toward knee).

Treatment/ Teaching   Bedrest. Elevate leg or affected limb. Moist hot packs or heating pad to area. Do not rub or massage area. Be seen by MD.

Refer to MD   For evaluation and treatment

Emergency   Sudden dyspnea, chest pain

Cross Reference   Calf Pain, Pulmonary Embolus

Acute exacerbation of hyperthyroidism, usually in known thyroid client

Etiology Infections, unusual emotional stress, any condition requiring emergency surgery

Assessment Very rare; usual symptoms include fever, tachycardia, weakness, tremor, extreme irritability, delirium, and coma.

Treatment/ Teaching Arrange emergency transportation to hospital.

Refer to MD

Emergency Emergency transportation to hospital

Cross Reference Hyperthyroidism, Hypothyroidism, Thyroid Replacement Therapy

Use of medication to increase thyroid-hormone level in body

Etiology　Remedy for hypothyroidism

Assessment

Treatment/ Teaching　Clients may experience symptoms of hyperthyroidism after starting treatment. Reassure client that symptoms are result of cumulative effect and will take a few days to subside after readjustment of medication. Have client call MD.

Refer to MD　If symptoms not subsiding

Emergency

Cross Reference　Hyperthyroidism, Hypothyroidism, Thyroid Crisis

Syndrome marked by brief attacks of severe pain in the distribution of 1 or more branches of the trigeminal nerve (jaw, eyes, forehead, cheeks)

Etiology Unknown

Assessment Intense pain is characteristic, usually described as stabbing, lightning-like, or shooting along distribution of 5th cranial nerve. Onset usually in middle or late life; incidence higher in women. Frequency of attacks varies from several times daily to several times a month or year. Attack may last from 1 to 2 minutes or as long as 15 minutes.

Treatment/ Teaching Analgesics usually not helpful due to sporadic nature of pain. No specific home treatment helpful.

Refer to MD For evaluation and management of pain

Emergency

Cross Reference Facial Pain

A blood-sucking acarid parasite

Etiology Usually picked up by brushing against low vegetation

Assessment Furuncle-like lesion containing a tick, usually pruritic

Treatment/ Teaching Attempt to pull tick out with tweezers and gentle traction. If head does not come out, it will fester and come out later. Try Vaseline to smother ticks and cause them to back out. A cloth soaked in acetone (nailpolish remover) and applied to tick loosens it in 10 minutes.

Refer to MD If client has been in area where Rocky Mountain Spotted Fever is endemic, or if fever and generalized illness follow appearance of tick

Emergency

Cross Reference Itching

Guidelines for interpreting results of test

Etiology

Assessment

Treatment/ Teaching

For clients with PPD reaction who are unable to report in 48 hours, have them draw circle around erythema present at 48 hours and come in for reading as soon as possible.

Positive reaction: Induration (not just redness) of 10 mm or more in diameter indicates past or present infection. The skin test becomes positive 2 to 8 weeks after infection with tubercle bacillus.

Negative reaction: Induration less than 5 mm in diameter.

Doubtful reaction: Induration of 5 to 9 mm, may be due to very recent infection, cross sensitivity to nontuberculous mycobacteria, or partial anergy (disappearance or marked decrease in the tuberculin reaction in the presence of a tuberculous infection).

Conversion reaction: A positive reaction that has developed within a year after a known negative reaction. It implies recent infection and is an important finding because the risk of developing clinical disease is greatest during the first 1 to 2 years after infection. Local policy may require reporting conversion reaction to Public Health Department.

Refer to MD

If known exposure to Tb or conversion reaction (client may need x-ray and Tb prophylaxis)

Emergency

Cross Reference

Guidelines to follow in evaluating postoperative course for tonsillectomy and adenoidectomy clients

Etiology

Assessment

**Treatment/
Teaching**
Slight oozing will occur initially; should stop within 24 hours, then area should remain dry. Surgical site of tonsillectomy appears white in color when healing. Ear pain is common up to 10 days post-op.

Refer to MD
If temperature 101° or over, if fever lasts longer than 48 hours post-op, or for ear pain accompanied by fever

Emergency
Active bleeding from surgical site

**Cross
Reference**
Blood in Vomitus, Sore Throat

Traumatic removal of a tooth, i.e., tooth knocked out

Etiology   Trauma

Assessment

Treatment/ Teaching   Do not remove any membranous material adherent to root. Be seen by dentist quickly (within 30 minutes). Attempt to replace the avulsed tooth into its socket prior to going to the dentist. If this is impossible, or if client is a young child, place tooth in cup of saline (¼ tsp salt to 1 cup water) and send with the client to the dentist.

Refer to MD   For evaluation of associated injuries

Emergency   Emergency visit to dentist

Cross Reference   Dental Problems

Systemic illness seen most commonly in menstruating females, characterized by high fever, chills, diffuse macular rash, vomiting, diarrhea, hypotension, desquamation

Etiology Probably caused by staphylococcus aureus toxin liberated in the bloodstream from a localized infection (i.e., vaginal tampon causing vaginal abrasions) or prolonged tampon use (more than 4 hours between changes)

Assessment Differentiation from systemic viral illnesses is difficult and dependent on obtaining menstrual history and history/pattern of tampon use.

Treatment/ Teaching To reduce risk of TSS, client should never leave tampon in more than 4 hours at a time. Do not use super-absorbent tampons; alternate tampons with pads.

Refer to MD If menstruating female with high fever, fainting, vomiting, diarrhea, rash

Emergency Hypotension in addition to above symptoms

Cross Reference Diarrhea, Fainting, Nausea, Rash, Vomiting

Guidelines for (and recommended) medications to be taken along

Etiology

Assessment

Treatment/ Teaching

Prescription medications prn: **tetracycline** 250 mg, 1 or 2 qid prn dysentery; Benadryl 25 mgm, 1 or 2 to every 4 to 6 hours prn allergic reaction; **Chloroquin** if client going into rural area where malaria is endemic (check with health department).

Nonprescription medications prn: Pepto Bismol in large doses for diarrhea;

Eat in first class restaurants or where food preparation habits are known. Avoid raw fruits and vegetables that cannot be peeled or cooked. Drink only bottled beverages or those made with boiled water (e.g., coffee, tea). Brush teeth with bottled water.

Refer to MD

To obtain prescriptions

Emergency

Cross Reference

Etiology

Assessment

**Treatment/
Teaching**

Refer to MD

Emergency

**Cross
Reference** Hyperthyroidism, Shakiness

TRICHOMONAS

Protozoal infection of lower reproductive tract

Etiology Trichomonas vaginalis

Assessment Usual symptoms consist of frothy, fetid, yellow-green vaginal discharge, irritation and itching of the vulva and vagina.

Treatment/ Teaching Cold compress to vaginal area prn irritation. Vinegar douche may be used, but not within 24 hours of being seen. Drug of choice is Flagyl (alcohol use is contraindicated during course of this drug). Both sexual partners need treatment. Use condom during course of treatment when having sexual intercourse.

Refer to MD For diagnosis and treatment

Emergency

Cross Reference Vaginal Itching, Vinegar Douche (Glossary)

A circumscribed area of erosion in the stomach or duodenum

Etiology   Hypersecretion of gastric acid, increased emotional tension and psychologic stress, tumor

Assessment   Burning epigastric distress on an empty stomach or 45 to 60 minutes after meals or nocturnal pain; relieved by food, antacids, or vomiting. Check for time pain occurs relative to eating and if antacids or eating relieve symptoms.

Treatment/ Teaching   If symptoms are stress related, use measures to reduce stress. Avoid coffee, tea, alcohol, ASA, chocolate, fatty or fried foods. Check stools for blood (dark, tarry color); note consistency.

Refer to MD   For steady abdominal pain unrelieved by home treatment

Emergency   Signs of active internal bleeding

Cross Reference   Abdominal Pain, Black Stools, Blood in Vomitus, Blood in Stools, Chest Pain, Nausea and Vomiting, Rectal Bleeding

Tissue breakdown secondary to pressure, commonly called a bedsore

Etiology Impaired blood supply and poor tissue nutrition due to prolonged pressure over boney or cartilaginous prominences

Assessment Ulcer begins with skin redness that disappears on pressure; skin and underlying tissues are still soft. This is followed by induration with a cyanotic tint or vesicle formation on the overlying skin. Finally, there is tissue necrosis. Destruction may be extensive, sometimes with exposure of bone.

Treatment/ Teaching Use of rings is contraindicated since they cause vasoconstriction to tissue surrounding affected area and can further impair circulation and healing. Treat early lesions with topical antichafing powder (e.g., baby powder, cornstarch). Gentle massage to affected area may help stimulate circulation. Use sheepskin, egg-crate mattress to reduce irritation and moisture and allow air to circulate around skin. Frequent change of position.

Prevention: Maintain adequate nutrition and skin hygiene. Keep linens and skin clean and dry. Turn bedfast, paralyzed, moribund or listless clients frequently (every hour) and examine for early breakdown of skin.

Refer to MD For treatment of open lesions and/or infection and necrosis

Emergency

Cross Reference Paralysis, Wound Infection

An acute catarrhal infection of the respiratory tract, usually with major involvement of the nose and throat

Etiology   Virus

Assessment   Differentiate acute from chronic process, presence of secondary infection. Determine if client is pregnant.

Treatment/ Teaching   Duration of symptoms is usually 4 to 10 days. ASA prn temp 101° and above (some degree of fever is useful in fighting infection). Decongestants (e.g., Dimetapp, Actifed) prn congestion in nose and sinuses. Expectorants (e.g., Benylin, Robitussin, 2/G) prn cough. Clear fluids. Rest. Saline nose drops. Vaporizer, steamy bathroom, or steam breathing over sink. Honey-lemon cough mix.

Refer to MD   For prolonged fever (beyond 48 hours); green, bloody, or bright yellow sputum or nasal discharge; prolonged cough, ear involvement, or sore throat (beyond 48 hours); chest pain; associated conjunctivitis not relieved by home treatment; wheezing; if pregnant

Emergency

Cross Reference   Antipyretic Drugs, Asthma, Bronchitis, Chest Pain, Cold Symptoms, Conjunctivitis, Cough, Earache, Fever, Honey-Lemon Cough Mix (Glossary), Influenza, Nasal Congestion, Pleurisy, Pneumonia, Saline Nose Drops, Sinus Congestion, Sinus Infection, Sore Throat, Swollen Glands, Wheezing

Presence of significant number of microorganisms in any portion of the urinary tract

Etiology   Majority of cases are caused by fecal flora of the coliform group of gram-negative bacteria (Escherichia, Enterobacter, Klebsiella, Enterococci, Pseudomonas, and Proteus).

Assessment   Classic symptoms include frequency, urgency, burning and pain, often chills and fever, nausea and vomiting, lassitude, generalized myalgia (especially in the low back). Most bacterial infections occur in women, sometimes related to sexual activity.

Treatment/ Teaching   Fluids, especially cranberry juice because of its acidity; avoid coffee, tea, coke (they act as bladder irritants). Urinary analgesics (e.g. Pyridium and Urised) help relieve burning; they do not act on the infection (Pyridium will turn urine orange. Urised will turn urine blue.). Heat to back prn pain. Urinating after intercourse, wiping from front to back may help in prevention. Urine sample for culture and sensitivity prior to any antibiotics.

Refer to MD   For treatment of UTI: client needs to be seen same day in most cases

Emergency

Cross Reference   Abdominal Pain; Back Pain; Bed Wetting (Peds); Blood in Urine; Burning on Urination; Pain in Side; Foley Catheters; Incontinence; Nausea and Vomiting; Nocturia; Prostatitis; Urine, Dark; Urine, Decreased Stream or Output; Urine, Excessive Output; Voiding Difficulty

Dark red or brown urine

Etiology   Infection, dehydration, drugs, bleeding in urinary tract

Assessment   Rely on history and ancillary symptoms. Check if person has recently eaten beets. Check for signs of dehydration and/or urinary tract symptoms.

Treatment/ Teaching   If asymptomatic and no trauma, force fluids.

Refer to MD   For symptoms of infection, trauma, dehydration, painless hematuria

Emergency   Gross hematuria, severe pain

Cross Reference   Bleeding After Urethral Dilatation; Blood in Urine; Burning on Urination; Dehydration; Hepatitis; Kidney Stones; Prostatectomy, Post-op; Urinary Tract Infection

Interference with the usual output of urine

Etiology Dehydration, retention, UTI, renal disease, prostatitis, surgery, recent catheterization, trauma, stones

Assessment Rely on history and ancillary symptoms.

Treatment/ Teaching Try urinating in warm tub bath if condition is due to retention and/or recent catheterization. Increase fluids without caffeine.

Refer to MD If no relief with home treatment, history of renal disease, prostatitis, UTI, mild trauma, or if severely dehydrated

Emergency Severe pain, anuria, severe trauma

Cross Reference Bladder Pain, Foley Catheters, Kidney Stones, Prostatitis, Urinary Tract Infection

Dramatic increase in urine output

Etiology Increased fluid intake, especially coffee, tea, alcohol; diuretics, diabetes, stress, urinary tract infection, prostatitis, renal tubular disorders, hypokalemia, hypercalcemic states (e.g., hyperparathyroidism)

Assessment Rely on history and ancillary symptoms.

Treatment/ Teaching If diabetic, symptom may indicate client is not under control.

Refer to MD For evaluation and treatment

Emergency

Cross Reference Diabetes Mellitus, Urinary Tract Infection

Any inflammation of the uveal tract (iris, ciliary body, and choroid of the eye)

Etiology   Unknown; may be part of underlying systemic disease

Assessment   Usual symptoms include pain, photophobia, circumcorneal inflammation. R/o conjunctivitis, acute glaucoma, and corneal ulcer.

Treatment/ Teaching   **Acute attack:** See an ophthalmologist

Chronic problem: Warm packs and analgesics (ASA or acetaminophen)

Refer to MD   For evaluation of acute attack or if episode more severe than previous attacks (if chronic problem)

Emergency

Cross Reference   Eye Pain, Iritis

Active, bright red or dark bleeding from the vaginal opening

Etiology Menstruation (normal and abnormal), abortion, placenta previa, abruptio placentae, ectopic pregnancy, intrauterine pathology (e.g., polyps, fibroids, carcinoma, endometriosis), PID, postpartum hemorrhage, uterine perforation (due to IUD), constitutional disorders (e.g., leukemia, purpura), emotional causes, infection in uterus or fallopian tubes

Assessment Determine if client is pregnant, postpartum, having menstrual period (with normal or abnormal flow); presence of abdominal pain, fever.

Treatment/ Teaching See individual cross reference cards.

Postpartum: Check for signs of infection (fever, foul-smelling vaginal discharge, abdominal or vaginal pain).

Postabortion: Bleeding for 3 days in decreasing amounts is normal. Check for increased bleeding, abdominal pain, fever, firm fundus.

Refer to MD For 1 episode of increased bleeding, bleeding unaccompanied by shock, signs of infection; if client is saturating a regular size pad in 2 hours or less, or bleeding is heavier than a normal menstrual period, client to be seen same day. If bleeding heavier than a normal menstrual period for more than 8 hours

Emergency Severe abdominal pain, lightheadedness, if pregnant, shock, uterine hemorrhage

Cross Reference Abortion, Abruptio Placentae, Ectopic Pregnancy, Menorrhagia, Menstrual Problems, Pelvic Inflammatory Disease, Placenta Previa, Spotting

Itching of the vaginal, vulvar, and/or perineal areas due to irritation or infection

Etiology Faulty feminine hygiene; tight, nonabsorbent clothing; leukorrhea; urinary incontinence; vaginitis; dermatitis; allergy or sensitivity reaction (e.g., ectopic eczema or contact dermatitis); systemic disease (diabetes mellitus, jaundice, Hodgkin's disease, uremia)

Assessment Rely on history and ancillary symptoms.

Treatment/ Teaching Oral antihistamines (e.g., Benadryl, CTM) for allergic reactions. Keep area clean; use bland, unscented soaps; avoid commercial feminine hygiene products or douches, **deodorant** tampons, and sanitary napkins. Carefully blot area dry to minimize irritation. Wear panties with a cotton crotch. Tepid sitz baths or cool compresses. Vinegar douches. Dusting powders of plain talc or cornstarch. No calamine or phenol compounds.

Refer to MD For evaluation and treatment

Emergency

Cross Reference Herpes, Genital; Trichomonas; Vaginal Yeast Infection

Guidelines to follow after a surgical vaginal repair

Etiology

Assessment   Check for increased erythema, drainage, fever, or increased tenderness.

Treatment/
Teaching   If unable to void, try warm shower or bath, glass of wine.

Refer to MD   If unable to void after home treatment and/or signs of infection present

Emergency

Cross
Reference

Infection of vaginal area

Etiology Candida albicans

Assessment Usual symptoms include pruritis and/or soreness in vaginal area; white, creamy, curd-like vaginal discharge (not purulent or offensive in odor). Often seen in clients with diabetes mellitus or those on antibiotic therapy or birth control pills.

Treatment/ Teaching Vinegar douche (do not use 24 hours before exam). Cold compresses to vaginal area or oatmeal bath to reduce itching. Use of tampons may reduce itching. Use cotton underpants instead of nylon. No vaginal deodorants, sprays, or medicated douche solutions. Sex partner should wear condom.

Refer to MD For diagnosis and treatment

Emergency

Cross Reference Oatmeal Bath (Glossary), Vaginal Itching, Vinegar Douche (Glossary)

Dilated, tortuous, superficial veins usually in the lower extremities

Etiology   Heredity, prolonged standing or heavy lifting, pregnancy, obstructive and valvular damage, fistulas

Assessment   Pain or discomfort secondary to arthritis; nerve root pressure of arterial insufficiency should be distinguished from symptoms associated with coexistent varicose veins.

Treatment/ Teaching   Support pantyhose, good walking shoes. Avoid prolonged standing or sitting with legs crossed. Elevate legs several times during the day, flex toes. Avoid constricting garments and knee-high hose.

Refer to MD   For evaluation and treatment

Emergency

Cross Reference   Calf Pain

Guidelines for evaluating postoperative course of vasectomy

Etiology   Surgical excision of part of vas deferens

Assessment   Mild, tolerable swelling is normal. Hematuria is an abnormal finding.

Treatment/ Teaching   Lie on back with towels to elevate scrotum for 24 hours, then out of bed with supporter. Ice pack to scrotum prn swelling and discomfort (client may have hematoma).

Refer to MD   See quickly for sudden swelling and intolerable pain and/or fever

Emergency

Cross Reference   Birth Control Methods, Testicle Problems

VENEREAL WARTS (Condyloma Acuminatum)

Common, benign epithelial tumors, usually transmitted sexually

Etiology Papovirus

Assessment May simulate syphilitic condylomatas; may proliferate and coalesce to form sizable plaques. Scattered warts may be seen within the vagina or rectum and may "seed" the skin around the orifice. Can appear anywhere on the genitalia, in the urethra in males, or in the rectal area.

Treatment/ Teaching

Refer to MD For topical treatment and/or surgical excision

Emergency

Cross Reference Penile Lesion, Syphilis

Impaired ability to see

Etiology Foreign body, injury, cataracts, carotid artery syndrome, papillitis, chorioretinitis, intraocular perforation, retinal detachment, diabetic retinopathy, glaucoma

Assessment Rely on history and ancillary symptoms.

Treatment/ Teaching **For foreign body:** Flush eye with tepid water for 10 minutes. See cross reference card.

Refer to MD If minimal symptoms or chronic condition

Emergency Sudden onset and/or eye pain

Cross Reference Eye, Foreign Body; Eye Pain; Eye Trauma; Glaucoma

Difficulty in urination

Etiology   UTI, prostatitis or prostatic enlargement, phimosis, trauma, renal stones or other obstruction of urinary tract, retention, genital herpes

Assessment Rely on history and ancillary symptoms.

**Treatment/
Teaching**
Retention: Attempt to urinate in warm tub bath

Genital herpes: Cold compresses to perineum prn

Refer to MD For infection, trauma, retention unrelieved by home treatment, obstruction

Emergency   Anuria, severe pain

**Cross
Reference**   Bladder Pain; Herpes, Genital; Kidney Stones; Prostatitis; Urinary Tract Infection

Etiology

Assessment

**Treatment/
Teaching**

Refer to MD

Emergency

**Cross
Reference** Nausea and Vomiting, Toxic Shock Syndrome

Viral lesion on skin or mucous membranes

Etiology   Virus

Assessment   Rough-surfaced, skin papule; plantar warts occur on soles of feet, are painful, callous-covered

Treatment/   Avoid touching warts; do not scratch. May use Compound W. Ice packs prn pain after wart
Teaching   removed with liquid nitrogen. Anogenital warts can be transmitted venereally.

Refer to MD   For treatment and/or removal of warts

Emergency

Cross   Venereal Warts
Reference

Breathing that is somewhat labored and with an audible whistling sound on expiration

Etiology Bronchial narrowing, bronchospasm, acute left ventricular failure, local bronchial obstruction (e.g., carcinoma, inflammatory stenosis, foreign body)

Assessment Rely on history and ancillary symptoms. Wheezing as a symptom of ventricular failure will be accompanied by associated signs of congestive heart failure. Check for history of chronic versus acute problem and degree of respiratory distress.

Treatment/ Teaching Clear fluids; vaporizer, steamy bathroom, or exposure to cool, damp night air. Bronchodilator medicines if already prescribed for asthmatic client.

Refer to MD For mild to moderate wheezing unrelieved by home treatment, if this is first known episode; for foreign body aspiration unaccompanied by other signs of respiratory distress

Emergency Severe respiratory distress

Cross Reference Allergic Reaction, Allergy Shot Reaction, Asthma, Choking, Congestive Heart Failure, Cough, Emphysema, Pulmonary Edema, Upper Respiratory Infection

Infestation of the body, usually the GI tract, by worms

Etiology   Ingestion of contaminated vegetation, shellfish, raw fish, water, meat

Assessment   Rely on history and visualization of worms; history of travel to tropical areas. Symptoms depend on type of worm and location involved.

Intestinal: Diarrhea, pain, signs of obstruction

Skeletal muscle: Abdominal pain, skin eruptions, neurologic signs

**Treatment/
Teaching**   Save stool specimen/vomitus for identification of worm type. Zinc oxide to rectal area prn itching.

Refer to MD   For diagnosis and treatment

Emergency

**Cross
Reference**   Pin Worms

Inflammation of an open lesion

Etiology   Bacteria

Assessment   Check for localized swelling, inflammation, purulent drainage, tenderness, swelling and tenderness of adjacent lymph nodes, presence or absence of fever, presence of systemic symptoms, appearance of red-streaking radiating away from wound. Determine etiology of wound.

Treatment/ Teaching   Evaluate need for tetanus immunization. Keep area clean and open if possible; dressing if drainage present. Moist hot packs to encourage localization and drainage.

Refer to MD   For evaluation and treatment with antibiotics if febrile, if red streaking is present, if no resolution with hot packing, if client has systemic symptoms, if purulent discharge present

Emergency

Cross Reference   Abrasion; Bee Sting; Bites, Animal and Human (Peds); Burns; Cellulitis; Laceration; Wound Infection, Post-op

Inflammation occurring at a recent surgical site

Etiology   Bacteria

Assessment   Check for increased erythema, purulent or serous drainage, red streaking away from incision, fever, increased tenderness or soreness.

Treatment/   Hot packs to area for 20 minutes, 4 times a day
Teaching

Refer to MD   If client febrile; for purulent drainage or red streaking

Emergency

Cross   Fever
Reference

PEDIATRIC
HEALTH
PROBLEMS

Information to be obtained

1. Name of client; phone number where the client will be located for the following 48 hours
2. Age
3. Chief complaint, other concerns
4. When was the child last well?
5. History of behavior since the child was last well, including activity, alertness, feeding pattern, fluid intake, sleep pattern, whether the child is lethargic or irritable, and a list of any medications the child is taking.
6. Presence or absence of fever
7. History of exposure to illness
8. What has been done to alleviate the child's symptoms? Has it helped? Note any change in routine or diet or if any medications have been given
9. History of medical problems, either resolved or ongoing

Factors affecting the decision to see a physician

1. Younger children: their symptoms can be vague and can change rapidly.
2. Persistent illness unresponsive to home treatment
3. Underlying chronic illness (e.g., diabetes) or a history of recurrent illness (e.g., otitis).
4. How "sick" the child seems to be
5. Level of anxiety displayed by caller

Home Treatment

1. Give **specific** instructions; have the caller repeat the directions back to be sure that they are understood.
2. Be certain that the caller has the equipment, medicine, time, and ability to carry out the instructions.
3. Advise the caller of **specific** indications to call back and when to call back.
4. Make plans for the parent or caller to be recontacted.

Discomfort in the abdominal area

Etiology   Infection in abdomen or elsewhere, constipation, injury, anxiety, obstruction, inflammation, basilar pneumonia, umbilical or other hernia, tumor

Assessment   Determine onset, if the pain is acute or chronic, the location (does it change?), if pain is persistent or intermittent, the degree of severity, relationship to feeding, if pain awakens child. Note other symptoms (e.g., vomiting, diarrhea, constipation, fever, headache, sore throat, cough or cold symptoms, urinary symptoms, anxiety), history of injury.

Treatment/ Teaching   Warm bath or heat to abdomen for 20 to 30 minutes. Clear fluid diet. Call back if pain unrelieved by heat; if pain increases in severity; is associated with tense, rigid abdomen; or if urinary symptoms, high fever, bloody emesis or stool, or persistent vomiting develop.

Refer to MD   For severe, constant, localized pain, especially if interfering with child's activity or causing child to cry; tense rigid abdomen; history of trauma; urinary symptoms; high fever; bloody emesis or stool; persistent, severe cough with fever

Emergency   Significant injury, shock, discolored and/or painful scrotum, umbilical hernia, passage of "currant jelly stools" (a large, formed blood clot)

Cross Reference   Clear Fluids (Glossary), Diarrhea, Urinary Problems, Vomiting

Guidelines for evaluating swelling in the abdominal area

Etiology Infection, obstruction, liver disease, kidney disease, hernia, trauma, hemorrhage

Assessment Determine the onset, duration and location of swelling; if child is uncomfortable; presence of discoloration or tenderness, vomiting, diarrhea, constipation, urinary retention, fever; history of trauma or similar episodes.

Treatment/ Teaching

Refer to MD Any acute abdominal swelling should be seen since it may indicate intestinal blockage, liver disease, hemorrhage, kidney disease, or tumor; most of the time it will be gastroenteritis, but this is difficult to distinguish by telephone.

Emergency

Cross Reference Abdominal Pain, Umbilical Cord Care

Rash that sometimes accompanies ampicillin or amoxicillin therapy

Etiology   Thought to be an interaction between the medication and viral illness.

Assessment   The appearance of the rash is variable; it is an erythematous, maculopapular rash anywhere on the body, often including the palms and soles. It is not pruritic and usually occurs toward the middle or end of a course of ampicillin or amoxicillin. Differentiate from an allergic rash.

Treatment/ Teaching   No treatment necessary. The rash will often persist for several days after the ampicillin or amoxicillin is discontinued. The decision to discontinue the medication should be individualized.

Refer to MD   If differentiation of rash is necessary

Emergency   Signs of allergic reaction, especially respiratory distress

Cross Reference   Allergic Reaction (Adult), Hives (Adult), Rashes

Guidelines for use and dosage

Etiology

Assessment

There is an association, but not yet a proved causal relationship between the use of aspirin in viral illnesses and subsequent Reye's Syndrome. Until this relationship is definitely established by the FDA, DO NOT recommend aspirin as the antipyretic agent of choice in viral illnesses, especially influenza and chickenpox (use acetaminophen) in persons under the age of 16.

Aspirin (ASA) is indicated for treatment of fever, pain, and inflammation. A common side effect is gastric distress.

Acetaminophen is indicated for treatment of pain or fever; it has no antiinflammatory effect. There are no significant side effects when given in therapeutic doses. Liver damage can result from overdosage.

CAUTIONS: Aspirin is excreted in the urine so a child with vomiting or poor liquid intake can become overdosed if the drug is given repeatedly. Children under 1 year of age should be given aspirin cautiously because they can easily receive a toxic overdose.

Treatment/ Teaching

Drug	How Supplied	Dosage
ASPIRIN (acetylsalicylic acid) May cause gastric distress **Use:** fever, pain, anti-inflammatory effect; always encourage extra fluids	Tablet: 1½ gr (80 mgm), 5 gr (325 mgm)* Suppository: 125 mgm, 200 mgm, 300 mgm	0-6 months: ½ gr (30 mgm) only on specific MD instructions or one time only with immunization 6-12 months: ½ gr (30 mgm) q4-6h prn 1-10 years: 1 gr (60 mgm) per year of age q4-6h prn

*Some "superstrength" preparations contain 7.5-10 gr per tablet. Have caller read the label to determine tablet size.

Treatment/ Teaching continued

Drug	How Supplied	Dosage
ACETAMINOPHEN (Tylenol, Datril, Liquiprin) No side effects in the proper dose; overdose may cause liver damage. **Use**: fever, pain; always encourage extra fluids	Tablet† Liquid†	10-15 mg/kg q4-6h; not to exceed 5 doses in 24 hours

Age		Wt	Dose
0-3	months	6-11 lb	40 mg
4-11	months	12-17 lb	80 mg
12-23	months	18-23 lb	120 mg
2-3	years	24-35 lb	160 mg
4-5	years	36-47 lb	240 mg
6-8	years	48-59 lb	320 mg
9-10	years	60-71 lb	400 mg
11-12	years	72-95 lb	480 mg

†Each brand name may have a different dosage strength. Have caller read you the label to determine dosage.

Refer to MD To pediatrician for use of these meds in infants under 6 months of age

Emergency Overdose of either medication

Cross Reference Crying and Irritability, Fever, Ipecac Protocol, Reye's Syndrome, Teething

Urine incontinence at night or during sleep

Etiology   Physiologic immaturity (child under 7 years old), urinary tract infection, emotional problem, metabolic disorder (e.g., diabetes), structural disorder (e.g., urethral valve weakness), inflammation (e.g., urethritis), neurologic disorder (e.g., meningomyelocele)

Assessment   Determine the child's age; if this is a new symptom in a previously bladder-trained child; if pain, frequency, or bloody urine is present. Sudden enuresis in a child who previously demonstrated control may be an early clue to urinary tract infection or diabetes. Usually therapy and/or urologic evaluation is not indicated unless the child is over 6 years old. Enuresis occurs normally until that time. However, the caller should discuss this with the primary physician. Children with school and learning problems commonly have enuresis.

Treatment/ Teaching   Ask if the child is a very deep sleeper. Consider use of a bell-ringing device that goes off at the time of voiding (e.g., Wee Alert—available at Sears). Reward the child verbally and possibly with a "gold star" on his calendar for dry nights. Avoid negative reinforcement such as scolding, diapering, or punishment. Giving the child the option of cleaning up or not cleaning up his bed helps to identify the problem as belonging to him.

Refer to MD   For evaluation and treatment

Emergency

Cross Reference   Blood in Urine (Adult), Urinary Problems

Guidelines for evaluating and treating bite injuries

Etiology

Assessment   Determine how the bite occurred (provoked or spontaneous), appearance of the bite (i.e., if the skin is broken), where bitten, size of wound, how deep, and if the wound is dirty or clean. What kind of animal? location of the animal?

Treatment/ Teaching   Wash wound well with soap and water, rinse. Ice pack or cold compress for swelling for 24 hours, then switch to heat. Come in for suturing within 4 to 6 hours of the injury if suturing required; MD may opt not to suture except facial wounds. Facial wounds need to be seen. Watch for signs of infection; cat scratches and human bites are likely to get infected more quickly than other animal bites. Report the incident to Animal Control prn. Cats and dogs should be observed for 2 weeks for signs of rabies. Bat and skunk bites must be reported to the Health Department. Check current tetanus immunization.

Refer to MD   For suturing, for secondary infection, if wound is on the face, if a rabid animal (e.g., bat or skunk) is suspected. If previous tetanus immunization but no booster in the past 5 years, refer within 72 hours of injury for booster. If no previous tetanus immunization, refer immediately.

Emergency   Massive tissue damage, hemorrhage

Cross Reference   Abrasion (Adult), Ice Pack (Glossary), Lacerations, Rabies (Adult), Tetanus Immunization, Wound Infection (Adult)

Guidelines for breast-feeding babies

Etiology

Assessment

Determine if there is a problem.

Treatment/ Teaching

Feeding Time

1) The baby will need help at first in finding the nipple and learning to nurse properly. Gently stroking baby's cheek next to the breast will encourage infant to turn toward the breast. Guide the nipple into baby's mouth by pressing the thumb above and 2 fingers below the nipple. (Never squeeze baby's cheeks or hold head and push it toward the breast; this may confuse and anger baby.)

2) Successful breast-feeding cannot take place if the baby's nose is stuffy. Teach mother to instill saline nosedrops, then gently aspirate nostrils before feeding if infant is congested.

3) Keep the breast from pressing against the baby's nose since this interferes with breathing. If baby does not grip the nipple firmly, gently press up under the chin with your thumb.

4) When baby is sucking properly, the entire brown area around the nipple will be in baby's mouth. If infant has just the nipple in his mouth, s/he will get very little milk and the nipple may become irritated.

Baby's Feeding Pattern

At first there will not be sufficient milk to satisfy the baby. Allow infant to nurse at each breast for 3 to 5 minutes; this will stimulate a larger milk supply. Colostrum will be present for the first 2 or 3 days and will be replaced gradually by milk. After the milk is fully established, the nursing period should not exceed 20 minutes, and not be more often than every 2 to 2½ hours. Breast-fed babies may need a vitamin mixture from 6 weeks on. Check with child's MD.

Treatment/ Teaching continued

Mother's Diet

1) If the mother is a pure vegetarian, her infant may not receive adequate nutrition.
2) While nursing, eat a well-balanced diet and drink plenty of liquids. Eat a great many fruits, vegetables, and eggs, with 2 servings of meat or fish daily.
3) Certain foods eaten by the mother can be passed through her milk and may cause discomfort to the baby (e.g., chocolate, garlic, spices, dark wheat, and vegetables of the cabbage family). One cause of colic in infants is the mother's overconsumption of cow's milk and cheese.
4) Mother should not take any medication unless prescribed by the MD; however, she should continue to take one-a-day multivitamin throughout the entire breast-feeding period.
5) For successful breast-feeding, it is essential for the mother to have plenty of rest.

Refer to MD

If baby is refusing all intake persistently, for projectile vomiting, respiratory distress, lethargy, irritability; if nipples become cracked, red, overly tender, or infected

Emergency

Cross Reference

Breast Infection (Adult), Colic, Spitting-Up

Redness, blistering or charring of the skin and deeper tissues caused by heat, electricity, flame, friction, or radiation

Etiology Accidental or intentional

Assessment Determine how the child was burned, extent and location of burn, appearance of burned area (e.g., red, blistered, charred, white), respiratory status, pulse, presence of shock.
Consider possibility of child abuse.

Treatment/ Teaching Immediately cool with water (not ice), i.e., soak in cool water, cold shower, or clean wet sheet. May use Bacitracin or Garamycin ointment on minor burns. ASA prn pain.

Refer to MD For any burn covering greater than 5% of the body surface and other than first degree. Wrap in clean sheet and transport.

Emergency Extensive burn or client in shock

Cross Reference Burns (Adult), Child Abuse or Neglect, Electric Shock (Adult), Shock (Adult)

CANKER SORES (Aphthous Stomatitis)

Small, very painful ulcers on the inside of the lips and throughout the mouth

Etiology Trauma, herpes, associated with illness, idiopathic

Assessment Determine the number of ulcers, presence of fever (if multiple ulcers, may have associated fever; otherwise, fever may be due to another illness). Check for history of irritant (e.g., vigorous brushing), foreign object, acid irritation (e.g., ASA or vitamin C tablets held in mouth). Check intake and state of hydration. Differentiate from herpes lesions. The first episode of herpetic stomatitis often results in multiple ulcers.

Treatment/ Teaching ASA or acetaminophen if multiple lesions causing discomfort. **Do not give ASA if viral etiology is suspected**. Swab lesions with Gly-Oxide. Saline mouthwash. Chloraseptic spray, Cepacol. Do not use viscous xylocaine (impairs gag reflex). Bland foods, not salty or acidic. Increase fluid intake. Dip Q-tip in baking soda and apply to lesion prior to meal (decreases pain and aids oral intake). Swish mouth out or gargle with Benadryl-Maalox mix (has a topical anesthetic effect). Expect lesions to last 7 to 10 days, regardless of treatment.

Refer to MD For poor intake or dehydration

Emergency

Cross Reference Aspirin and Acetaminophen; Benadryl-Maalox (Glossary); Dehydration; Herpes Simplex (Adult); Saline Mouthwash (Glossary); Canker Sore (Adult)

A mild but highly contagious disease characterized by the appearance of vesicles on skin and occasionally the mucous membranes

Etiology   Varicella virus (Herpesvirus varicellae)

Assessment   Fever and malaise appear prior to eruption of vesicles. Rash is most prominent on face, scalp, and trunk, is papular changing to vesicular, pustular, and finally crusting; rash is pruritic. Incubation period is 14 to 20 days.

Treatment/ Teaching   Fluids. Acetaminophen prn fever and itching. Baking soda baths. Calamine lotion to rash. Antihistamines orally to manage itching. Loose, light-weight clothing. Trim fingernails short, wear sox on hands at night if scratching. Keep client isolated until pox have crusted (about 7 days from onset of rash).

Refer to MD   For secondary infection or complications (but generally avoid bringing the client into a setting that exposes others); if accompanied by increasing cough and rising fever, client must be seen to rule out chickenpox pneumonia.

Emergency   If immunosuppressed or immunodeficient (i.e., cancer client, client on steroid therapy) **and** is exposed to or develops chickenpox, the client must be seen.

Cross Reference   Aspirin and Acetaminophen, Fever, Itching, Rashes, Baking Soda Bath (Glossary)

Guidelines for handling child abuse in a telephone encounter

Etiology   Most people who abuse their children were also abused as children.

Assessment   Approximately 10% of alleged accidents in children under age 6 are due to physical abuse.
                    Estimates of the usual age for child abuse: one-third occur under 1 year of age; one-third from
                    ages 1 to 3; and one-third over age 3. Injuries frequently associated with abuse include burns
                    (when the pattern does not match the history given); fractures (especially chip fractures of long
                    bones); subdural hematomas (secondary to shaking injuries); whipping with a belt or electric
                    cord; hair-pulling with scalp hematoma; ear twisting, resulting in ecchymosis in the ear; rup-
                    tured tympanic membrane from ear boxing; retinal hemorrhage; multiple abrasions, fractures,
                    and bruises in various stages of healing; cigarette burns, dunking burns, slap marks on cheek.
                    Child abuse should at least be considered with any of the following medical problems: skin
                    bruises, soft tissue swellings, fractures, dislocations, tender extremities, burns, head injuries,
                    subdural hematomas, unexplained seizures or comas, malnutrition problems, or "crib deaths."

Treatment/   Some parents may call before abusing the child and indicate they have reached their frustra-
Teaching   tion tolerance. These parents should not be put off. Listen to them and provide initial counsel-
                    ing, crisis intervention prn. Determine if this is an ongoing problem. Refer for mental health
                    counseling as appropriate. Advise parent to bring the child in for medical evaluation if abuse is
                    suspected. DO NOT INDICATE TO PARENTS THAT ABUSE IS SUSPECTED. Rather,
                    notify emergency room personnel to be aware of possible abuse situation.

Refer to MD   For evaluation of injuries and possible hospitalization

Emergency   Child comatose, severely injured, or dead

Cross   Burns, Fractures or Dislocations (Adult), Genitalia Problems
Reference

Paroxysmal fussing, most common from 4 pm to 10 pm

Etiology May be related to irritability, irregular gastrointestinal peristalsis, and other, as yet unintegrated, functions characteristic of the first 2 to 3 months. In breast-fed babies, it may be directly related to the amount of cow's milk protein the mother ingests. Babies on formula may also be affected by type or amount of milk intake.

Assessment Usually occurs in infants under 3 months of age. Attacks are usually sudden in onset, often in afternoon or evening. During more intense attacks baby will flex thighs against the abdomen or rigidly extend them. Crying is more or less continuous. Feet may be quite cold. The infant does not respond to usual measures used for comfort, but may be relieved with the passage of feces or gas. The infant is frequently difficult to burp after the feeding that preceeds the attack. Colic must be differentiated from other causes of fussiness. Ask about feeding patterns, weight loss, fever, lethargy, vomiting, and stool pattern.

Treatment/ Teaching Hold baby upright. Burp baby. Place infant prone across lap or across warm water bottle on lap and gently rock child. Do not overfeed. Use rhythmic motion (e.g., rocking, car ride, carrying baby in front pack). Use a pacifier, soft music, quiet environment. If all else fails, put baby down in a quiet, safe place and take a break from trying to quiet baby. (This gives parents a respite and may keep tension from escalating to a point where abuse may occur.) Parents need sympathy, understanding, and reassurance that colic will resolve at about 3 months. They need to be relieved of their guilt over a fussy baby and be counseled to avoid yelling at each other because the baby is crying.

If breast-feeding: Ascertain amount of milk and milk products the mother is eating. Advise decreasing mother's dairy intake (no more than 8 to 12 oz of milk in 24 hours is necessary). Urge other fluids, especially water. Good general diet for mother. If no change in colic, mother can resume milk intake.

If bottle-feeding: Try reducing total amount of baby's milk intake, replacing with other fluids. Observe for improvement. If no change in colic, resume previous feeding and check with pediatrician.

Refer to MD If colic severe, if medications needed (e.g., antispasmodics); if suspect a medical problem is cause of fussiness

Emergency Passage of "currant jelly" stool (classic symptom of intussusception)

Cross Reference Abdominal Pain, Breast-Feeding, Crying and Irritability, Feeding of Infants

COMMON COLD (Upper Respiratory Infection)

Guidelines for treating a common cold in children

Etiology Virus

Assessment Determine presence of fever, cough, or difficulty in breathing (e.g., presence of wheeze or stridor, etc.), feeding or sleeping difficulty, presence of ancillary symptoms (i.e., earache, sore throat, appearance of discharge). Also determine onset and duration of illness, if other family members show similar symptoms.

Treatment/ Teaching Elevate head of bed. Cool mist and vaporizer. Increase clear liquid intake, dilute juice, etc. Older infants often refuse solids and should be allowed to take **liquids only** while ill. Acetaminophen (**no ASA**) if over 6 months for discomfort and fever. Saline nose drops. Use bulb syringe to clear infant's nasal passages. Decongestants (e.g., Sudafed, Dimetapp) in older children; not necessary in infants. Have parent check back by telephone for sudden high fever, respiratory distress.

Refer to MD For high fever or breathing difficulty; earache; persistent sore throat (over 48 hours duration); or thick, purulent (yellow or green), or bloody discharge from nose

Emergency Severe respiratory distress

Cross Reference Aspirin and Acetaminophen, Cough, Croup, Earache, Saline Nose Drops (Glossary), Sore Throat, Wheezing

Hard, infrequent stools passed with difficulty

Etiology   Inadequate fluid intake, diet, intestinal obstruction

Assessment   Determine the frequency, color, consistency of stool; presence of blood, stomach cramps, vomiting, abdominal distention, fever. Determine what food and fluids are currently in the diet, if the child is satisfied (and gaining weight if breast-fed).

Treatment/ Teaching

Infants: Breast-fed babies will often have a soft, yellow stool only every 6 to 10 days and this is **normal**. Babies normally strain passing a bowel movement. Give Karo water (1 tbsp **dark** Karo in 3 oz water) or Karo formula once daily as a laxative prn. Have mother repeat the directions to ensure that the correct proportions have been understood. Do not overdose with Karo solution. No enemas, suppositories, or laxatives (dangerous to newborns). In bottle-fed babies, determine exactly how the formula is being prepared. Incorrect preparation (i.e., too strong formula) is a common cause of infant constipation. If suspect inadequate intake is cause, suggest supplement and weight check at clinic. If infant on juice, may give prune or apricot juice.

Children: Increase fluid intake, especially water and fruit juice (prune or apricot). Decrease milk intake to 1 pint daily. Eat cooked fruits, particularly prunes, apricots. Include bran cereal, vegetables, salads in diet.

Refer to MD   If symptomatic constipation present (crying, bloating, vomiting, hard bloody stools); if no response to home treatment

Emergency   Signs of obstruction

Cross Reference   Abdominal Pain, Diarrhea, Vomiting

Etiology

Assessment

**Treatment/
Teaching**

Refer to MD

Emergency

**Cross
Reference**　　**Adult**: Gamma Globulin Information, Hepatitis, Mononucleosis, Mumps, Rubella, Scarlet Fever or Scarlatina

Pediatric: Chickenpox, Fifth Disease, Measles, Roseola, Strep Throat

A sudden expulsion of air from the lungs, accompanied by an explosive noise resulting from opening the glottis

Etiology Irritation of the upper airway due to colds, postnasal drip, allergy, foreign body, asthma, croup; dry environmental air, smoke (especially from wood stoves)

Assessment Determine the nature of the cough (i.e., wet or dry), sudden or persistent, occurring day or night or both; associated symptoms (e.g., congestion, fever, sore throat, earache, chest pain, abdominal pain, presence of hemoptysis); history of allergies or asthma; possible aspiration of a foreign body; presence of respiratory distress (e.g., stridor, wheeze, grunting, retracting, increased rate, cyanosis). Cough that occurs during exercise may suggest exercise-induced asthma. Choking-type cough that occurs abruptly suggests a foreign body.

Treatment/ Teaching Elevate head of bed. Clear fluids; avoid dairy products. Honey-lemon cough mix if child over 1 year of age (use corn syrup instead of honey if child under 1 year old; may put mixture in a cup of tea that is supersaturated with sugar; give in small amounts). Use cool mist vaporizer. In naturally cool, moist environments, open the window and lower the environmental temperature. Use commercial cough syrups if over 1 year of age.

Wet cough: Use a decongestant (e.g., Sudafed).

Dry cough: Use an expectorant during the day and a cough suppressant at bedtime (e.g., Benylin, 2/G, Cheracol D.)

Allergy: Use an antihistamine/decongestant (e.g., Actifed, Dimetapp).

Asthmatic: Check if child is taking usual asthma medications and if they are offering relief of symptoms. Explain why cough is important (to clear the airway, to bring up phlegm).

Refer to MD For suspected foreign body, cough associated with high fever, cough persistent over 2 to 3 weeks

Emergency Respiratory distress, tachypnea, persistent stridor, significant wheeze

Cross Reference Common Cold; Croup; Foreign Body, Swallowed; Honey-lemon Cough Mix (Glossary); Pediatric Doses of Commonly Used Medications; Wheezing

An acute illness characterized by inspiratory stridor and barky cough

Etiology   Virus

Assessment   Most commonly affects children between 3 months and 3 years of age, and characteristically occurs during the late fall and early winter. The onset is gradual, with a history of several days of symptoms of upper respiratory tract infection prior to the sudden onset of barking cough, usually at night, then inspiratory stridor. There are generally only mild elevations of temperature and the child does not appear toxic. If the lower respiratory tract is significantly involved, wheezing is present.

Non-serious croup: Tends to respond promptly to steam or cool, moist air, gets better in daytime, but worse at night and in the early morning hours.

Serious croup: Gets relentlessly worse and does not respond well to steam or cool, moist air. Determine gradual vs sudden onset. Differentiate from epiglottitis, which has rapid onset of high fever, respiratory distress, drooling, loss of phonation, difficulty swallowing, and is an emergency.

Treatment/ Teaching   Listen to child breathe over the phone. Cool mist vaporizer or take child out in cool, moist night air; if these options are not available, sit with child in steamy bathroom. Urge clear fluids, popsicles, ice chips. Ice collar to neck. Honey-lemon cough mix (if over 1 year) may be helpful or 2/G for older child. No decongestants (they are drying and may exacerbate croup). Prophylactic dose of acetaminophen (**no ASA**), at hs and 4 hours later to keep temperature down. Call back if increasing distress or unresponsive to steam.

Refer to MD   If no improvement with vaporizer, if continuous stridor present, or if unable to retain fluids

Emergency   Drooling, difficulty swallowing, fighting for air, cyanotic, high fever; child looks extremely ill or toxic

Cross Reference   Cough, Epiglottitis, Honey-Lemon Cough Mix (Glossary), Ice Collar (Glossary), Wheezing

Symptoms indicative of discomfort or displeasure

Etiology Colic, teething, tiredness, excess intestinal gas, fluid or infection in middle ear, undetected fever, hunger, meningitis, intussusception, any kind of infection, trauma

Assessment Determine presence or absence of fever, child's activity level (lethargic vs pursuing usual activities), presence of swollen gums and/or drooling, history of URI or otitis, any sign that child is pulling or rubbing at his ears, recent changes in eating, drinking and/or sleep patterns, any history of injury, how "sick" the child appears to the mother, presence of any other ancillary symptoms (e.g., vomiting, diarrhea, bulging fontanel).

Treatment/ Teaching Burp, hold, and comfort infant. Aspirin or acetaminophen in appropriate dose if over 2 months of age (**no ASA if virus suspected**). Warm water bottle to infant's abdomen. Observe for further symptoms and call back if other symptoms develop or fussiness persists.

Refer to MD If child appears "sick" to mother (especially infant under 6 months); if febrile, intermittently lethargic, not eating, not vigorous; if suspect significant medical problem (i.e., meningitis, acute abdomen, otitis, injury, infection, or obstruction)

Emergency Projectile vomiting; extreme lethargy; child seems to have severe pain

Cross Reference Aspirin and Acetaminophen, Ear Infection (Adult), Feeding of Infants, Meningitis (Adult), Teething

Negative fluid balance in body; fluid intake too low to replace fluid loss

Etiology   Vomiting, diarrhea

Assessment   Determine quantity and type of fluid intake, amount and frequency of vomiting and/or diarrhea within past 6 to 8 hours. Determine frequency and quantity of urine output (is diaper damp or completely saturated?).

Treatment/
Teaching   Child needs to be seen if urine output is less often than every 6 to 8 hours, if mucous membranes pale and dry looking, eyes sunken and/or if child very lethargic. Infants can dehydrate very rapidly. For minimal symptoms with no vomiting, increase clear fluids (especially Gatorade or Pedialyte), until normal urine output resumes.

Refer to MD   For evaluation and possible hospitalization

Emergency   If shocky or unresponsive

Cross
Reference   Diarrhea, Vomiting

Irritation on the buttocks and perineum, secondary to urine, stool, or infection

Etiology Irritation, yeast infection, staphylococcal infection, contact dermatitis, eczema, seborrhea

Assessment Usual symptoms include erythema and thickening of the skin in the perineal area. In 80% of cases of diaper dermatitis lasting more than 4 days, the affected area is colonized with Candida albicans even before the appearance of the classical signs of beefy red, sharply marginated dermatitis with satellite lesions. Determine appearance, distribution, duration of the rash, what is being used on the skin; how diapers are laundered; if plastic pants are being used; and if the rash appears elsewhere on the body. Ask if the mother had a vaginal yeast infection during or before pregnancy and if the child has been on any recent antibiotic therapy.

Treatment/ Teaching Change diapers frequently (check hourly for wetness) and immediately after a bowel movement. No plastic pants; remove waterproof cover of disposable diapers. Expose baby's bottom to air and sunshine as much as possible. Wash diapered area with warm water prn. Occasionally use a little mild soap (e.g., Ivory, Baby Castile). If yeast suspected, encourage adding plain yogurt or acidophillus milk to diet. Discontinue all use of bubble baths, bath oils. Do not put fabric softeners or other additives in the laundry.

Diaper rinse: To help neutralize the strong ammonia fumes of urine, add 2 cups of vinegar to final rinse water when laundering diapers. When buttocks can't be open to the air (or at nap or bedtime), use soothing and protecting ointments (e.g., Desitin, A&D, Diaperene), or simply a liquid corn oil or shortening from the kitchen. Cornstarch **should not** be used since it is a medium in which Candida albicans flourishes.

Refer to MD For rash that is not improving with home treatment; if pustular rash develops (may need specific cream, i.e., Nystatin with or without hydrocortisone, to combat yeast infection)

Emergency

Cross Reference Rashes

An increase in the frequency and liquidity of stools

Etiology Viral or bacterial infection, obstruction, food allergy, malabsorption, campylobacter, Yersinia, Giardia

Assessment Rely on history and ancillary symptoms. Determine number of stools, onset and duration, consistency, color, size when started, presence of blood or mucus, state of hydration, intake of fluids, i.e., what, how much, recent change in diet.

Cause	Age	Fever	Characteristics of Stool and Associated Symptoms
Milk intolerance	Over 5 days	None	Stools often streaked with blood or mucus. Nasal congestion. Fussiness to hard crying. Often family history positive for milk allergies.
Starvation	10 days-2 months	None	Small, frequent, watery, greenish stools. Seen in breast-fed infants. Poor weight gain.
High gluten (wheat) ingestion in mother	10 days-10 months	None	Large, bulky nonformed stools with pungent odor, often with mucus. Found in breast-fed babies.
High gluten ingestion in infant	6 months-2 years and over	None	Same as above. Occurs in infants when teething biscuits, graham crackers, or high protein cereal is introduced.
Virus	3 months and older	Present or absent	Often watery, no particular odor. Often preceded or accompanied by vomiting; may be mildly explosive. URI symptoms may be present.
Pathogenic (Shigella, Salmonella, E. coli)	Any age, but often toddler	Often high with shaking chills; may be preceded by convulsion	Explosive; mucus and blood present. Crying. Close contacts may have same symptoms. May have been around turtles, water fowl at edge of lakes, or eaten undercooked fowl.

Assessment continued

Cause	Age	Fever	Characteristics of Stool and Associated Symptoms
Giardia	Any age, but usually preschoolers and children in day care	Often	Chronic watery or bulky stools. Weight loss, abdominal discomfort.
Malabsorption	Any age	Often absent	Chronic weight loss.

Treatment/ Teaching

Discontinue all solids, foods, and milk except for breast milk. Offer only Pedialyte or Lytren to infants. Over 1 year, Gatorade, flat 7-Up or ginger ale, water, or weak tea may be given in small amounts (1 to 2 oz) as often as the child will take them for 24 hours.

Infant: Advance to ½ strength soy formula (i.e., diluted with twice as much water as can calls for). Gradually increase to full strength soy formula over 24- to 36-hour period. No solids.

Infant or child: In addition to above, add nonsweetened cereal (rice or corn), meats, ripe bananas for 1 to 2 days. Then slowly add vegetables (yellow) and (later) fruits. No cow's milk or other dairy products for 4 to 5 days after diarrhea stops, then start skim milk (not boiled). Continue soy formula during these 4 to 5 days. If diarrhea restarts, back up 1 step. Call back if vomiting or dehydration develops, diarrhea persists, or if steady severe abdominal pain.

Milk allergy: Use saline nose gtts to clear the nostrils. Differentiate between this and neonatal Shigella by history (did mother have diarrhea) and by culture. Try soy formula.

Starvation: Increase frequency of breast-feeding or formula.

High gluten ingestion, mother: Discontinue eating wheat products.

High gluten ingestion, infant: Discontinue teething biscuits, graham crackers, high protein cereal, and other wheat products.

Virus: If breast-fed, increase frequency of feedings. Supplement with Pedialyte or Lytren. Discontinue formula, cow's milk, and/or other solids. Substitute Pedialyte in children under 10 months, or Gatorade for older infant. Proceed as per above routine regarding adding solids and formula.

Pathogenic bacteria (Shigella, Salmonella, E. coli): Careful hand washing and handling of soiled linens.

Refer to MD

Needs to be seen based on urgency of symptoms. If dehydrated; if liquid stools persisting despite treatment; if stools bloody, black, or white; for high fever, listlessness, severe abdominal pains

Emergency

Cross Reference

Abdominal Pain, Dehydration, Vomiting

Pain in or around ear

Etiology   Trauma, impacted wax, internal or external infection, eustachian tube dysfunction

Assessment

Cause	Pain	Fever	Associated With
Trauma	Variable, increased when pinna moved	None	History of trauma
Impacted wax	Same as above	None	Past history of same
External otitis	Same as above	None unless severe	Swimming or impacted wax
Eustachian tube dysfunction	Worse when supine or going up in altitude	Usually none or low grade	Postotitis, diving, swimming, sinus infection, post-URI, taking bottle to bed
Viral otitis media	Often excruciating but self-limiting, 2 to 4 hours	None or low grade to medium	URI, rhinorrhea. Serosanguinous fluid may leak from ear; usually self-limiting, no emergency.
Bacterial otitis media	Often persistent and severe; may be dull; infants very irritable and bat at ears; may look toxic.	Moderate to high	URI, sinusitis, nasal rhinorrhea or congestion. Mucopurulent fluid may leak from ear; no emergency, but child must be seen.

Treatment/ Teaching

Trauma: Cold compress or ice pack initially, then follow with heat.
Impacted wax: Warm oil drops, e.g., liquid shortening, Colace, or Ceruminex (1 application only), followed by gentle irrigation.
External otitis: ASA prn pain until seen.
Eustachian tube dysfunction: Instillation of medicated nose drops (Neo-Synephrine) or saline.
Viral otitis: Acetaminophen (**no ASA**) prn pain, saline or medicated nose drops (e.g., Neo-Synephrine). Warmth to ear. May use ½ to 1 tsp cough syrup containing codeine 1 time prn severe pain. Check for allergy: most codeine cough syrups contain 8 to 10 mg per tsp.
Bacterial otitis: Same as viral; must be seen. Children with PE tubes will more commonly have drainage with viral or bacterial infections. See within 24 hours, sooner if severe pain or fever present.

Refer to MD   For evaluation of earache (how soon depends on the severity of pain and discomfort, degree of fever and toxicity, severity of trauma)

Emergency   Severe trauma, toxic; to rule out serious infection such as meningitis

Cross Reference   Aspirin and Acetaminophen, Common Cold, Crying and Irritability

Etiology

Assessment

Treatment/ Teaching

Refer to MD

Emergency

Cross Reference   Eczema (Adult)

Inflammation of the epiglottis resulting in acute respiratory distress

Etiology   Bacteria

Assessment   Generally affects children between the ages of 3 and 7 years, with no particular seasonal distribution. Must not be confused with viral croup. Onset is abrupt over a period of only a few hours. Young children often present with high fever and respiratory distress; older children may appear toxic and, in addition, complain of difficulty swallowing and severe sore throat. Because of extreme dysphagia, pooling of secretions in the posterior pharynx and drooling are prominent signs. The child may have muffled voice but not be hoarse; within a few hours after onset of symptoms, may be in marked respiratory distress with severe inspiratory stridor and retractions. Determine if onset sudden or gradual, degree of respiratory distress, presence of drooling or difficulty swallowing.

	Epiglottitis	**Viral Croup**
Common cause	Hemophilus influenzae	Parainfluenza virus; respiratory syncytial virus
Most common age range	Usually 3–7 years, but any age	Usually less than 3 years, but any age
Seasonal occurrence	None	Late fall, winter
Clinical onset	Rapid, acutely ill	Preceded by rhinitis and cough for several days
Dysphagia	Marked; may be drooling	None
Fever	Over 101°–103°F	Variable, usually less than 103°F

Treatment/ Teaching   Must be seen STAT if suspect epiglottitis. Keep child calm and upright. Nothing PO (may need a tracheostomy).

Refer to MD   Arrange for emergency transportation to hospital.

Emergency   Marked respiratory distress, drooling, dysphagia, toxic, aphonia, high fever

Cross Reference   Croup

Guidelines for treatment of these symptoms in children

Etiology   Blocked tear duct, allergies, viral or bacterial infection, foreign body

Assessment   **Blocked tear duct:** Usually presents as tearing and mucopurulent discharge from the eye in an infant.

Conjunctivitis: Tearing, mucus, redness, and swelling without pain or photophobia is usually a viral or bacterial conjunctivitis.

Allergic symptoms: Include itchy eye, redness, tearing without purulent drainage, lid and conjunctival swelling, and a history of allergies.

Orbital cellulitis: Lid redness and swelling, pain with pressure on globe often accompanied by fever, malaise, and prostration.

Uveitis: Pain, photophobia, or decreased visual activity.

Treatment/ Teaching   Cool, wet compresses. Antihistamine (e.g., CTM, Benylin) prn allergic symptoms. Check back if condition does not respond to treatment or if it worsens.

Refer to MD   Within 24 hours if symptoms are those of conjunctivitis; routine appointment for evaluation of blocked tear duct or recurrent allergic conjunctivitis

Emergency   Acute pain, redness, photophobia and/or seriously decreased visual acuity; lids bright red and swollen

Cross Reference   Conjunctivitis (Adult); Eye, Injury or Foreign Body; Uveitis (Adult)

Trauma to eye

Etiology   Blow or foreign body

Assessment   Determine how injury occurred and if the eye or just periorbital area is affected, if there is eye pain, redness, discharge, vision problem, diplopia, if pupils are equal. Determine if it feels like "there is something in the eye" and what the foreign body is.

Treatment/ Teaching   **Foreign body:** Flush eye immediately for 10 minutes with water or saline (saline hurts less than plain water).

Periorbital bruising: Cool compresses or ice pack.

Refer to MD   For marked periorbital swelling, bruising, eye pain, decreased visual acuity, photophobia, diplopia, disconjugate gaze, pupil inequality; if foreign body cannot be dislodged, if it feels like there is still "something in eye" after flushing or after dislodged by MD, or if cause of injury was chemical

Emergency   Sudden loss of vision, severe eye pain, hemorrhage from eye

Cross Reference   Eye: Infection, Inflammation, Allergic Symptoms

Guidelines to follow

Etiology

Assessment

Determine if mother is breast- or bottle-feeding the infant and if there is some problem. If by bottle, determine how the formula is being mixed, if solids are being given; if so, what kinds and in what quantity. If breast-feeding, check on maternal diet, drug ingestion, general health (if indicated).

Treatment/ Teaching

Birth to 6 months

Human breast milk is recommended as the only food in the infant's diet for the first half-year; it is "nature's perfect baby formula." Almost all babies will take the correct amount of breast milk on a "flexible demand" schedule. Commercial infant formula may be given as a supplement prn. Vitamin A, C, & D (with iron) drops may be given to breast-fed infants. Mothers on special diets might need vitamin supplements for themselves and their breast-fed infant.

Commercial infant formula (with iron) should be given if breast-feeding is not chosen or is discontinued. The formulas are made from cow's milk (e.g., Enfamil and Similac) or soybean protein (e.g., Isomil, ProsoBee, Soyalac); these are high-quality copies of human breast milk and nutritionally are very similar to it. Powder, concentrate, and ready-to-feed forms are the same nutritionally, but vary greatly in cost per feeding. Extra vitamins and iron are not needed. Most babies will take the correct amount of formula on a "flexible demand" schedule, but consult practitioner if baby takes more than 32 ounces (1 quart) of formula daily or shows inadequate weight gain.

Solid foods are best delayed until the infant is 6-months-old, because of the additional potential for food allergy and obesity. In the past, solids were introduced earlier, but there are no sound nutritional reasons for doing so.

Treatment/
Teaching
continued

Age 6 to 12 Months

Continuation of breast-feeding as the main source of nutrition is encouraged. Vitamin-iron supplement should be continued.

Commercial infant formula should be given as the primary nutritional source if breast-feeding is not done; cow's milk (skim, 2%, or whole) is not recommended during the 1st year.

Solid foods should be introduced gradually after 6 months of age. A customary sequence starts with rice cereal for 1 month and then slowly add new foods at 3 to 5 day intervals with fruits and vegetables first, followed by meats. "Finger foods" may be introduced at 8 to 12 months followed by selected table foods. If the home water supply has no **fluoride**, ask practitioner about a supplement.

Over 12 Months

Some infants continue to nurse, which is encouraged if it continues to be a satisfactory experience for both baby and mother; otherwise, switch to cow's milk and table foods. Additional vitamins are probably not necessary if the child takes a balanced diet. Irregular appetite and eating habits are typical for this age group. Like their parents, infants usually eat 3 to 6 times daily.

Refer to MD

If infant refusing all intake persistently; unable to feed because of other medical problems, i.e., respiratory distress, lethargy, irritability, projectile and/or persistent vomiting

Emergency

Cross
Reference

Breast-Feeding

Elevation of body temperature above normal (97° to 99° F, 36° to 37.5° C)

Etiology   Viral, rickettsial, bacterial, fungal, and parasitic infections (most common causes)

Assessment   Rely on history and ancillary symptoms. Determine if the client "acts sick" (is child playful, alert, fussy, lethargic?). Check the status of appetite, fluid intake, urine output. Determine presence of respiratory distress, history of medical problems (e.g., chronic disease, frequent otitis, febrile convulsions, recent immunization, exposure to illness), presence of symptoms that give clue to etiology; duration and level of fever; and what treatment has been given.

Treatment/ Teaching   Reassure that fever itself is not harmful unless over 105°F (40.5°C) and prolonged or if history of febrile convulsions; rather, fever is body's normal response against infection. Treatment of fever is more for child's comfort than because fever itself is dangerous. Rectal temperatures will usually register 1 degree higher and axillary temperatures 1 degree lower than oral temperatures. Dress child lightly, don't bundle. Aspirin or acetaminophen in dosage appropriate to age if temp 101°F or above. **Do not give ASA if viral etiology is suspected.** Combine aspirin and acetaminophen only if there is a history of febrile convulsion and child is less than 6 years old, if temperature is over 105°F (40.5°C), or if viral etiology is not suspected. Recheck temperature 1 hour after giving antipyretic to determine drug's effectiveness. **Never** use cold baths or alcohol sponges. Occasionally a lukewarm bath is helpful to slowly lower the child's temperature. Encourage fluid intake (children with high fevers can dehydrate). Recontact parents in 1 to 2 hours and then prn until illness resolves.

Refer to MD   For persistent fever without an explanation that lasts longer than 48 hours; for high temperature in young infant; if child appears "sick" (lethargic, irritable); if other symptoms indicate significant illness (e.g., otitis, pneumonia, meningitis); if any doubt, have child seen.

Emergency   Fever associated with repetitive seizures, loss of consciousness, severe respiratory distress

Cross Reference   Aspirin and Acetaminophen, Chickenpox, Dehydration, Immunization Reactions, Inguinal or Scrotal Swelling, Measles, Meningitis (Adult), Pediatric Doses of Commonly Used Medications, Roseola, Seizures, Strep Throat

FIFTH DISEASE (Erythema Infectiosum)

A mildly contagious childhood disease with a characteristic rash and usually no fever or other symptoms

Etiology Probably a virus

Assessment The rash is the only common feature and occurs in three stages: (1) rash appears on the face with intensively red eruption mainly on cheeks ("slapped face"), contrasting to pale area around mouth; (2) approximately 1 day later, red spots (maculopapular) appear on the extremities, first on extensor and then on flexor surfaces and trunk, as rash fades it becomes *lacelike*, lasts 1 to 2 days, up to 1 week; (3) after rash disappears, it may reappear up to 1 to 2 weeks later precipitated by heat, sunlight, cold, or taking a bath. Child usually does not feel ill or have any other symptoms.

Treatment/ Teaching None indicated; may return to school.

Refer to MD For evaluation if diagnosis is in doubt

Emergency

Cross Reference Rashes

Foreign body swallowed or blocking airway

Etiology   Accidental or intentional

Assessment   Determine what was swallowed, size, if object sharp, when object swallowed. Determine presence of respiratory distress, difficulty swallowing, drooling, vomiting or regurgitation, substernal or abdominal pain, blood in vomitus or stool, fever.

Treatment/ Teaching   **If child choking:** Try to open mouth and dislodge object with finger. If unsuccessful, lean child forward or suspend upside down and thump on back. If still unsuccessful, lean child forward or suspend upside down and squeeze abdomen firmly.

If asymptomatic: Observe child and call back if further symptoms develop. If sharp object swallowed, give bread product and milk to form spongy cushion and hopefully prevent perforation. If foreign body is meat without bones, give meat tenderizer as a paste.

Refer to MD   For substernal or abdominal pain, fever, blood in vomitus or stool, moderate symptoms after ingestion of foreign body

Emergency   Severe respiratory distress and unable to dislodge foreign body

Cross Reference   Choking (Adult)

Etiology

Assessment

**Treatment/
Teaching**

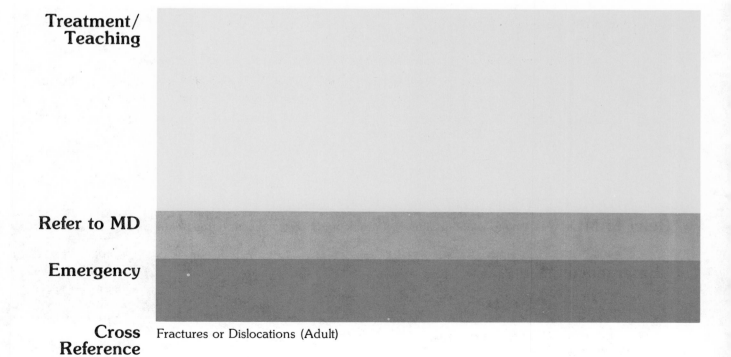

Refer to MD

Emergency

**Cross
Reference** Fractures or Dislocations (Adult)

Common problems of genital area in young children (primarily male)

Etiology Trauma, infection, foreign body

Assessment
1) **Contact dermatitis (balanitis):** Results from finger/penis contact after contact with an offending substance.
2) **Entrapment:** Pre-speech male infants may get a "hangman's noose" of scalp hair completely encircling the penis with attendant swelling and cutting.
3) **Penis caught in zipper.**
4) **Foul-smelling discharge:** Males: may be UTI or gonococcus. (If gonococcus, must r/o abuse). Females: vaginal foreign body most common cause. R/o UTI.
5) **Ulceration** of meatus (male) often secondary to penis rubbing against diaper. R/o closure of meatus versus inadequate meatus.

Treatment/ Teaching
Balanitis: If seen early, can be ameliorated rapidly with tapered (decreasing) steroid regimen; if seen late, may need antibiotics.

Entrapment: Find offending hair and cut with scissors if penis not too swollen.

Penis in zipper: Grease organ and zipper track with Vaseline and reverse zipper motion that originally entrapped the penis, or cut off bottom of zipper and pull edges apart.

Ulceration of penile meatus: Vaseline to tip of penis; change diapers frequently; open diaper area to air periodically.

Refer to MD For diagnosis and treatment if problem not resolved with home treatment or if urinary meatus closed

Emergency Extreme swelling, pain, anuria

Cross Reference Child Abuse or Neglect, Urinary Problems

Pain or discomfort in the head

Etiology Trauma, drugs, illness or impending illness (especially viral or strep), tension, migraines, infection, tumor

Assessment Determine onset, duration, severity, location of headache; history of similar episodes, presence of ancillary symptoms (fever, vomiting, rash, lethargy, irritability); history of predisposing factors (trauma, drugs, exposure to illness, family history of migraine).

Treatment/ Teaching Rest in darkened, quiet room. ASA or acetaminophen in appropriate dosage. Call back if headache persists or if other symptoms develop.

Refer to MD If recurrent problem, if unrelieved with home treatment, if associated with other serious ancillary symptoms

Emergency Altered state of consciousness, severe pain, if suspect meningitis

Cross Reference Aspirin and Acetaminophen, Head Injury, Meningitis (Adult)

Guidelines for evaluating trauma to head in child

Etiology Trauma

Assessment Determine how the injury occurred, distance of fall, surface material against which the impact occurred (falling 4 or more feet and striking the head against concrete is often associated with a skull fracture); any loss of consciousness, child's orientation, responsiveness, alertness, if vomiting present and if it occurred once or repeatedly, presence of headache unrelieved by ASA, extent of injury (areas of swelling, bruising, lacerations), reactiveness of pupils, presence of bloody or watery drainage from nose or ears. Determine extent of other injuries, if child on any medications, history of underlying medical problem (e.g., seizure disorder).

Treatment/ Teaching Observe neurologic signs for 24 hours (Head Injury in adult section). Awaken child every 2 hours to observe alertness, responsiveness, pupil reactivity and equality, ability to move all extremities. Cool compresses or ice pack to area of swelling. Light diet. Expect child to be mildly drowsy for a short time, to vomit once or twice, and to have some swelling and bruising at the site of the injury.

Refer to MD If severe fall or blow; loss of consciousness or memory or altered level of consciousness; lethargy, unsteady gait; if combative or confused; persistent vomiting or headache (unrelieved by ASA); for suturing or evaluation of other significant injuries; for blood or serous fluid leakage from ears or nose

Emergency If unresponsive or paralyzed (if paralyzed, don't move except under medical direction)

Cross Reference Head Injury (Adult), Lacerations, Lethargy, Vomiting

Etiology

Assessment

Treatment/ Teaching

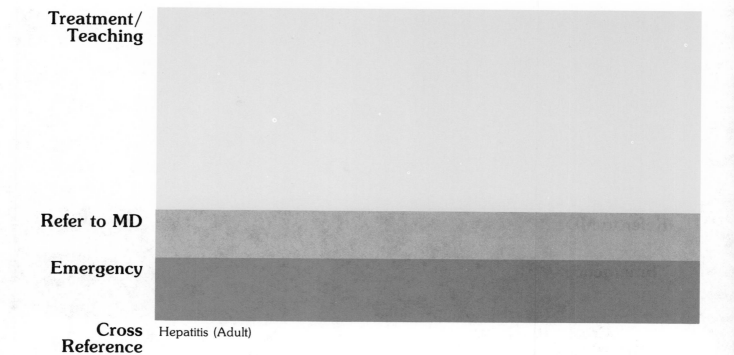

Refer to MD

Emergency

Cross Reference   Hepatitis (Adult)

Etiology

Assessment

**Treatment/
Teaching**

Refer to MD

Emergency

**Cross
Reference** Hives (Adult)

Schedule of recommended immunizations for children

Etiology

Assessment

**Treatment/
Teaching**

Age	Immunization
6 weeks	DPT1; OPV1 (bottle-fed babies)
4 months	DPT2; OPV1 (breast-fed babies)
9 months	DPT3; OPV2; Tine Test
15 months	MMR
2 years	DPT4; OPV3; Tine Test
5 years	DPT5; OPV4; Tine Test
Every 10 years	DT booster with Tb test

If older child is partially immunized, discuss need for further immunization with MD. Measles vaccine given before 12 months or before 1967 should be repeated. Pertussis should not be given over age 6. Rubella should not be given to pubertal girls unless it is certain that pregnancy will be avoided for 3 months after vaccine is administered. Smallpox is no longer given routinely. DT booster is given at the time of an injury or burn if it is more than 5 years since last booster and child has received initial series of 5 injections.

Refer to MD

If immunization status is unclear

Emergency

**Cross
Reference**

Bites, Animal and Human; Gamma Globulin Information (Adult); Immunization Information (Adult); Tetanus Immunization

Common reactions to immunizations

Etiology

Assessment

Treatment/ Teaching

DPT: May cause redness and swelling at the injection site and fever. Treat with ASA or acetaminophen and cool compresses. Reaction generally subsides in 24 to 48 hours. A firm lump may remain at the site for months.

Measles: Occasionally 5 to 12 days after vaccination child may have measles-like rash and fever lasting several days. Child is not contagious; cannot give measles to anyone from immunization reaction.

Rubella: Child may show occasional transient arthritis or arthralgia 2 to 4 weeks after vaccination.

Refer to MD

For exceptionally high fever or convulsions, deterioration of mental status

Emergency

Cross Reference

Fever, Immunization Information

Etiology

Assessment

**Treatment/
Teaching**

Refer to MD

Emergency

**Cross
Reference**   Impetigo (Adult)

Guidelines for evaluation

Etiology   Hernia, hydrocele, trauma, torsion, infection

Assessment   Determine location of swelling, if it is persistent or if it comes and goes; if area is red, tender, dark or bruised, tense. Determine onset, history of trauma, if child is uncomfortable, irritable, and if vomiting or fever is present. Hydrocele: A slow, painless, nondiscolored, nontender swelling of the testicle with a collection of water in the scrotal sac that usually resorbs slowly.

Treatment/ Teaching   **Hernia:** To help reduce it, soothe and comfort the child; often sitting in warm bath is helpful. May also place child in slightly head-down position and with heel of palm, exert gentle steady pressure on the hernia. Child may be seen routinely in clinic.

Hydrocele: Child may be seen routinely in clinic; reassure parent.

Refer to MD   If hernia cannot be reduced, if swelling comes and goes or is easily reduced

Emergency   Swelling that is acute, tense, tender, red or blue (could be torsion, infection, injury, or incarcerated hernia) or if scrotal swelling is irreducible especially if baby is irritable, vomiting, or febrile

Cross Reference   Fever, Swelling

Evaluation of trauma in children

Etiology   Accidents, falls, abuse

Assessment   Determine site of injuries, how trauma occurred, presence of active bleeding, respiratory status, pulse, color, state of alertness and responsiveness, presence of vomiting. Further questions depend on site and severity of injuries.

Treatment/ Teaching   Ensure adequate respirations and heart rate; CPR if necessary. Measures to avoid shock (keep child supine, warm, etc). Do not move child until certain there is no neck injury and possible extremity injuries are splinted. Direct pressure to active bleeding site.

Refer to MD   For injuries requiring treatment

Emergency   If unstable, shocky, for impaired respiratory or cardiac status, extensive injuries

Cross Reference   Burns, Child Abuse or Neglect, Fractures or Dislocations (Adult), Head Injury, Lacerations, Shock (Adult), Sprain (Adult), Strain (Adult)

Etiology

Assessment

Determine location and extent of swelling, type of insect, presence of generalized symptoms (i.e., hives, generalized swelling or facial swelling, dyspnea, generalized itching), history of allergic reaction to insect bites or stings.

Treatment/ Teaching

Cool compresses or ice pack for 24 to 48 hours prn swelling and itching. Remove stinger if appropriate (do not squeeze; flick out with fingernail). Swelling may be more prominent the 2nd day. Elevation of extremity will help decrease swelling. Calamine lotion, meat tenderizer (monosodium glutamate) poultice, or baking soda paste. If child over 1 year old, antihistamine (e.g., Dimetapp, Novahistine, Benylin, Benadryl, Actifed, Periactin) for discomfort or itching ½ to 1 tsp every 4 to 6 hours prn. Call back if symptoms of generalized allergic reaction or secondary infection appear.

Flea bites: Same local treatment; deflea pets and house.

Refer to MD

If generalized symptoms or swelling extending to major joints beyond bite; for signs of secondary infection

Emergency

Allergic reaction, anaphylaxis

Cross Reference

Allergic Reaction (Adult); Baking Soda Paste (Glossary); Bee Sting, Insect Sting (Adult); Meat Tenderizer Paste (Glossary)

Guidelines for use of Ipecac in treating selected poisonings

Etiology

Assessment

Treatment/
Teaching

Call POISON CONTROL CENTER _____ to see if Ipecac is indicated. If instructed to use Ipecac, remember, it does not work on an empty stomach. First give 6 to 8 oz of milk, water, juice, pop (nothing red). Then give 2 tsp of Ipecac for the child 8 months to 3 years; 3 tsp for child 3 to 5 years; 2 tbsp for adults. Next, give 1 to 2 more glasses of liquid and let child run around and play (speeds up action of Ipecac). If vomiting has not occurred in 20 minutes, pull the tongue forward and stroke back of tongue, offer more fluids. If vomiting does not occur within 5 minutes of stroking the tongue, repeat the Ipecac and liquid. If vomiting does not occur within 20 minutes after the 2nd dose of Ipecac, the child will have to be seen in the clinic or hospital.

Refer to MD

If no emesis after 2nd dose of Ipecac or in case of repeated vomiting after Ipecac dose, or if substance puts client at risk

Emergency

Toxic symptoms

Cross
Reference

Aspirin Overdose (Adult), Poison Ingestion (Adult), Poison Ingestion

Etiology

Assessment

**Treatment/
Teaching**

Refer to MD

Emergency

**Cross
Reference**   Itching (Adult)

Wounds with torn or ragged edges

Etiology   Trauma

Assessment   Determine how injury occurred, site, depth, and length of laceration, presence of active bleeding, motor or sensory impairment, function of adjacent organs, need for tetanus immunization.

Treatment/ Teaching   Pressure to site of bleeding. Ice pack to reduce bleeding and swelling. If suturing not required, clean with soap and water. Do not use iodine, hydrogen peroxide, or other caustic agents that could kill tissue and slow healing. May use antibiotic ointment (e.g., Bacitracin). Approximate edges of wound and tape edges together. Watch for signs of infection (indicate what they are). Lacerations of the tongue and mouth are usually due to tooth-bite; generally not sutured unless large or deep enough to be seen on outside of mouth or if bleeding continues. **CAUTION:** a tear or puncture injury in the throat or back of the mouth occurs when children bump sticks or toys held in the mouth. These can be serious and should **usually be seen**.

Refer to MD   For suturing (need to suture within 6 to 8 hours of injury), possible impairment of adjacent organ, motor or sensory dysfunction, persistent bleeding, need for tetanus booster (need to have had initial series and immunization within past 5 years)

Emergency   Extensive laceration, hemorrhage, extensive loss of motor or sensory function

Cross Reference   Ice Pack (Glossary), Tetanus Immunization

A condition of drowsiness, indifference, apathy, or sluggish inactivity

Etiology Normal component of many illnesses, head injury, ingestion of drugs or poisons, seizure disorder

Assessment Determine degree of lethargy (is child awake? responsive to parent's voice? able to recognize parent? able to eat and drink?) and activity (e.g., coloring, watching TV, running, riding tricycle). Is there a history of possible causes such as head injury, ingestion, infection, seizure?

Treatment/ Teaching Rest, if symptoms are expected with child's illness and are mild, or if part of postictal state and child has known seizure disorder (and if not instructed by MD to be seen after a seizure). Rest for 1 hour following a head injury if no other neurologic signs and child is responsive and easily aroused. Watch for increasing lethargy and/or appearance of other symptoms; have parent call back if these occur.

Refer to MD If child not responsive to voice, not oriented to place, does not recognize parent, or unable to eat or drink; if lethargy is increasing or accompanied by other serious symptoms

Emergency Comatose or recurrent seizures

Cross Reference Convulsions (Adult), Head Injury (Adult), Head Injury

Etiology

Assessment

**Treatment/
Teaching**

Refer to MD

Emergency

**Cross
Reference**   Lice (Adult), Pediatric Doses of Commonly Used Medications

An abnormal gait

Etiology Injury, viral inflammation of muscle or joint contents, arthritis, osteomyelitis

Assessment Determine onset and duration of limp, degree of discomfort, history of injury, localization of pain or tenderness, movement limitations in extremities, redness, bruising, swelling, fever, rash, history of musculoskeletal problems.

Treatment/ Teaching Rest. Elevation. Ice pack to reduce swelling. Splint during transport if there is a possible fracture or significant pain.

Refer to MD For evaluation of persistent limp or significant injury; see immediately for significant pain, high fever, well-localized pain, joint swelling, redness, heat, and tenderness.

Emergency

Cross Reference Fractures or Dislocations (Adult), Sprain (Adult), Strain (Adult)

A highly contagious, acute disease

Etiology Virus

Assessment Characterized by fever, cough, coryza, conjunctivitis, eruption (Koplik's spots) on the buccal or labial mucous membrane, a bright red exanthem on the mucous membrane of the nasopharynx, photophobia, and a spreading maculopapular cutaneous rash. Usual mode of transmission is by direct contact with droplets from the infected person; less commonly airborne. Incubation period is from 10 to 12 days, the child is contagious from the 5th day of the incubation period through the 1st few days of the rash. Rash may resemble roseola, scarlet fever, rubella, infectious mononucleosis, or drug eruptions. Generalized lymphadenopathy and sometimes splenomegaly may persist for weeks after acute illness and are often confused with infectious mononucleosis or leukemia.

Treatment/ Teaching Fluids. Acetaminophen prn fever (no ASA). Expectorant and decongestant (e.g., Benylin, CTM) for nasal congestion and cough. Light clothing prn fever. Darkened room prn photophobia. Calamine lotion to rash, baking soda bath prn itching. Bedrest during febrile period.

Refer to MD All cases should be seen for diagnosis; for treatment of secondary infection; for vaccination of exposed but unvaccinated infants or children or for gamma globulin for persons at risk

Emergency

Cross Reference Aspirin and Acetaminophen, Fever, Immunization Information, Rashes, Rubella (Adult), Baking Soda Bath (Glossary)

Etiology

Assessment

**Treatment/
Teaching**

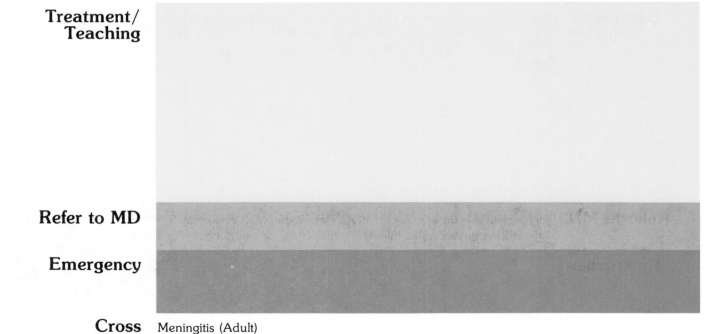

Refer to MD

Emergency

**Cross
Reference**   Meningitis (Adult)

Etiology

Assessment

Treatment/ Teaching

Refer to MD

Emergency

Cross Reference   Mumps (Adult)

Sanguinous drainage from nose

Etiology   Trauma, allergies, irritation of the nasal mucosa, bleeding disorder, nose-picking

Assessment   Determine if child or family member has history of unusual bleeding, bruising, allergies, frequent nosebleeds, recent trauma, upper respiratory infection, picking at nose.

Treatment/ Teaching   Sit erect, blow nose once to remove clots. Pinch nose firmly below boney portion between thumb and forefinger for at least 10 minutes. Use small ice pack at bridge of nose. After bleeding stops, sit quietly and erect for 15 to 30 minutes. Do not blow nose (this can disrupt clot). If above fails, soak small cotton plug with medicated nosedrops (e.g., Neo-Synephrine, Afrin) and insert into anterior nostrils (Do not use in presence of chronic illness or hypertension.); apply pressure for 10 minutes; leave cotton in for several hours.

Refer to MD   If no relief with home treatment, for evaluation of recurrent nosebleeds, or if history of bleeding disorder (e.g., leukemia, hemophilia)

Emergency   Hemorrhage from nose

Cross Reference   Nose, Broken (Adult)

PINWORMS (Enterobiasis)

Infestation of the colon with the pinworm

Etiology   Pinworm (Enterobius vermicularis), seatworm

Assessment   Symptoms include rectal or vaginal itching. The adult worms reside in the cecum and colon. The gravid females crawl out and deposit thousands of eggs in the skin folds of the anus, especially at night, causing intense itching. When the child scratches, the ova stick to the fingertips and under the nails and eventually get to the mouth and are swallowed, resulting in autoinfection. Contamination of clothes and environment leads to the infestation of fresh hosts; it is not unusual for several members of the same household to harbor pinworms. Determine if worms have been seen (they are white, about ½" long, and are best seen at night or early morning around the rectum). Use Scotch tape test to confirm. (Evert a strip of Scotch tape, gummed side outward, on the edge of a tongue blade, dab the perianal area at night or first thing in the morning to collect specimen for identification).

Treatment/ Teaching   A common problem; other family members may need treatment. Not an emergency. Vermox (dose is 1 chewable tablet per person); do not give to pregnant women or children under 2 years of age (use Pova for children under 2). Reinforce good hand washing, trim fingernails close and keep them clean. Wash infected bed linen and underwear in hot soapy water. Zinc oxide ointment to rectal area prn itching. Sitz bath with Epsom salt or large amount of table salt helpful for itching.

Refer to MD   For evaluation and treatment; if urinary symptoms present and infection suspected.

Emergency

Cross Reference   Urinary Problems

POISON INGESTION

Accidental or intentional ingestion of toxic matter

Etiology

Assessment   Determine substance ingested (brand name and ingredients listed on label), when ingested, amount ingested (i.e., original amount and how much was left), present condition of child, if evidence of substance on clothing, smell of it on breath, etc. Determine if Ipecac is available.

**Treatment/
Teaching**   Contact POISON CONTROL CENTER _____ for specific directions and information on the ingested substance. If Ipecac is clearly indicated and client is alert, see cross reference card on Ipecac Protocol. (Most fire stations have Ipecac if none readily available; also available at pharmacies and 7-11 stores.) **Do not** induce vomiting for hydrocarbons and oils (e.g., gasoline, kerosene, polishes, paint thinner) or for caustics (e.g., Draino, Lye, bleaches, detergents). With or without Ipecac, give child milk or water. Call pediatrician immediately and have family keep their telephone line open.

Refer to MD   If substance puts child at risk or harm; bring along container of ingested material, sample of ingested material, and bucket to catch vomitus.

Emergency   Child comatose, toxic, or in serious condition

**Cross
Reference**   Aspirin Overdose (Adult), Ipecac Protocol

Stenosis of the pyloric channel resulting from hypertrophy of the circular muscle

Etiology   Unknown

Assessment   Usual symptoms include vomiting (usually projectile), constipation, poor weight gain or weight loss, and dehydration. Vomiting usually begins between 2 to 4 weeks of age and progresses to projectile vomiting after each feeding; in about 10% of cases, it may start at birth. The vomitus does not contain bile but may be bloodstreaked. The infant is hungry and nurses avidly, but there is a decrease in the number and size of stools and failure to gain weight. The condition occurs in 1 out of 500 births; males are affected 3 to 4 times more commonly than females.

Treatment/ Teaching

Refer to MD   For evaluation of persistent vomiting, constipation, dehydration, fretfulness, lethargy

Emergency   Severe dehydration

Cross Reference

Etiology

Assessment

**Treatment/
Teaching**

Refer to MD

Emergency

**Cross
Reference**   Bites, Animal and Human; Rabies (Adult)

Skin eruptions

Etiology   Communicable disease, contact with chemicals or irritants, medications, allergens, unknown causes

Assessment   Determine location of rash, when it first occurred, the spread (where and how fast), current distribution, appearance (color, raised or flat, blister, pustule, crusted, wet or dry, confluent or separate lesions, petechial, purpuric or hemorrhagic), if rash blanches with pressure, shape and size of lesions, or pruritis. Are there associated symptoms (fever, sore throat, cough, headache)? recent exposure to illness, drugs, insect bites, allergens? history of similar rash?

Treatment/ Teaching   **For itching:** Cool bath with cornstarch or soda, antihistamine (e.g., Benadryl, CTM), Calamine lotion.

If allergic: Remove allergen, give antihistamine prn for urticaria (e.g., Benedryl, CTM), Calamine lotion.

If communicable disease: Keep comfortable, avoid exposure to well persons during period of communicability. See specific cross reference cards. Follow progress by phone.

Refer to MD   For sore throat and fever with fine rash; for localized, crusted, or weepy lesions (impetigo); pruritic, persistent and spreading rash (i.e., scabies vs allergy)

Emergency   Petechial or purpuric rash (doesn't blanch); generalized urticaria of rapid onset, especially with dyspnea; child toxic or has stiff neck

Cross Reference   Ampicillin/Amoxicillin Rash, Chickenpox, Cornstarch Bath (Glossary), Diaper Rash, Eczema (Adult), Fifth Disease, Hives (Adult), Impetigo (Adult), Measles, Ringworm (Adult), Roseola, Scabies (Adult), Scarlet Fever or Scarlatina (Adult), Seborrhea

Encephalopathy with fatty degeneration of the viscera

Etiology Unknown; viral agents such as influenza B, varicella, exogenous toxins, or intrinsic metabolic defects in urea-cycle enzymes are possible contributing factors. The use of ASA in viral illness may be associated.

Assessment Suspect Reye's in child with acute onset of encephalopathy without known heavy metal or toxin exposure. Usual signs include minor URI of short duration preceding onset of vomiting, irrational behavior, progressive stupor, and coma. Resolving chickenpox may be present in 10% to 20% of cases. Restlessness and convulsions may occur.

Treatment/ Teaching

Refer to MD For evaluation of vomiting following chickenpox or URI

Emergency Convulsions, progressive loss of responsiveness

Cross Reference Aspirin and Acetaminophen, Chickenpox, Common Cold, Pediatric Doses of Commonly Used Medications

A benign, self-limiting illness of early childhood characterized by a discrete pink rash following a febrile period

Etiology   Probably virus; no specific virus isolated

Assessment   The typical clinical picture is 3 days of sustained high fever (sometimes with a febrile convulsion at the onset) in a child who otherwise appears well. A discrete pink rash is the most characteristic finding. It typically appears as the fever decreases or shortly thereafter. The rash is occasionally generalized and may coalesce; it lasts as briefly as several hours, as long as 2 days. Usually occurs in children under 3 years of age.

Treatment/ Teaching   Acetaminophen (no ASA) for fever. Increase fluid intake. Light clothing and tepid bath to help reduce fever. Since diagnosis is usually late, it is unreasonable to isolate child during the presence of fever and rash because no secondary cases have been observed.

Refer to MD   For febrile seizure; for differential diagnosis of high fever before rash appears

Emergency   Sustained seizure activity, especially accompanied by respiratory distress

Cross Reference   Aspirin and Acetaminophen, Fever, Rashes

Etiology

Assessment

**Treatment/
Teaching**

Refer to MD

Emergency

**Cross
Reference** Scabies (Adult)

Etiology

Assessment

**Treatment/
Teaching**

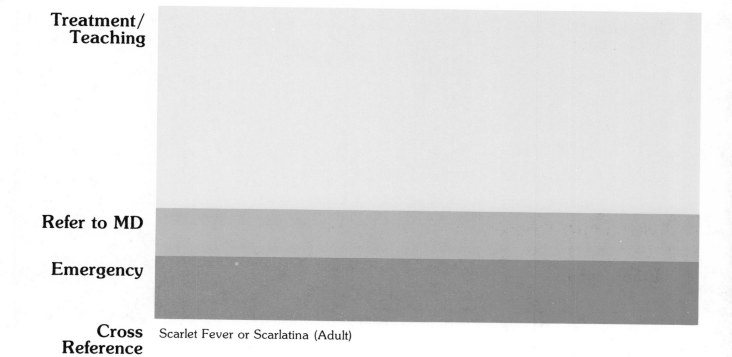

Refer to MD

Emergency

**Cross
Reference** Scarlet Fever or Scarlatina (Adult)

SEBORRHEA

Dermatitis accompanied by overproduction of sebum

Etiology Unclear

Assessment Seborrhea is an erythematous, scaly dermatitis accompanied by overproduction of sebum, and occurs in areas rich in sebaceous glands (face, scalp, and perineum). This common condition occurs predominantly in the newborn and at puberty, the ages of maximal hormonal stimulation of sebum production. It appears on the scalp as scaly and flaky, occasionally with yellow crusts. On skin it often appears in flexor creases, especially inguinal and behind ears; is moist, red, scaly, occasionally with yellow crusts. It is called "cradle cap" in newborns.

Treatment/ Teaching Frequent shampoos with medicated products (e.g., Sebulex, Selsun Blue, Sebuton). Treat skin with topical cortisone preparation. In infants, use baby oil to soften scales and loosen crusts ½ hour before shampooing, then scrub with soft brush and castile soap or baby shampoo. Repeat daily until condition improves.

Refer to MD For evaluation and management of chronic problem

Emergency

Cross Reference

Involuntary contraction of muscles, resulting from abnormal stimulation

Etiology Fever, head trauma, congenital malformations, infections, perinatal factors, epilepsy

Assessment If child is convulsing at time of call, give emergency directions immediately, then take history. Determine if there is a history of seizures or if current one is the 1st, if child is on any medication for seizures and if all doses have been taken, presence of fever or illness, recent trauma, use of drugs. Differentiate from syncope (in which child usually reports that "things went black" before "sinking" to the ground; tonic-clonic movements do not occur, consciousness returns as blood flow to brain increases, there are no postictal phenomena and usually no retrograde amnesia).

Treatment/ Teaching 1) Place client on flat surface, preferably on side (to prevent self-injury and aspiration); move furniture or objects prn. 2) Remove any food or foreign material from mouth (if possible) to prevent aspiration. 3) Expect drowsiness after seizure. 4) Don't bundle a child with fever. 5) Child with epilepsy should notify MD that s/he had another seizure. 6) Nothing PO while child is unresponsive. 7) Placing an object between the teeth usually is not necessary. Beware of putting fingers between teeth.

Refer to MD If 1st seizure, or if other symptoms warrant being seen

Emergency Client cyanotic, in respiratory distress, or if seizure does not stop spontaneously within 5 to 10 minutes

Cross Reference Convulsions (Adult), Fever

Inflammation of the pharynx

Etiology   Virus, bacteria, postnasal drip, mouth breathing

Assessment   Determine onset and duration of symptoms, presence of ancillary symptoms (URI, rash, pus on tonsils, swollen glands in neck), severity of pain, presence of respiratory distress. Differentiate from canker sores that cause pain with swallowing. Have parent inspect mouth, gums, tongue, and throat and describe.

Treatment/ Teaching   Increase fluid intake, especially cold beverages, ice cream, popsicles. Avoid acidic juices that might increase discomfort (e.g., orange or grapefruit). Aspirin or acetaminophen (no ASA if viral etiology) in dosage appropriate to age. Saline gargles or throat lozenges if old enough.

Refer to MD   For sore throat persisting beyond 48 hours, or if accompanied by fever or rash

Emergency   Acute respiratory distress, drooling, febrile, appears toxic

Cross Reference   Aspirin and Acetaminophen, Common Cold, Epiglottitis, Fever, Strep Throat

Regurgitation of a portion of a feeding

Etiology   Overfeeding, feeding too fast, inadequate burping, gastroesophageal valve incompetence

Assessment   Distinguish from vomiting. Determine the quantity, frequency, forcefulness of spitting up. Determine if onset is recent or if it is an ongoing problem, if baby is gaining weight, if child seems ill (has discomfort, fever, cough, diarrhea, URI, etc.).

Treatment/ Teaching   Many babies will spit or regurgitate nonforcefully several times a day, but still gain weight. These babies are well and usually outgrow symptoms when they begin to walk. Use infant seat while feeding, burp frequently. Elevate head of bed. Do not press on abdomen. Avoid overfeeding and feeding too fast. Thicken the formula.

Refer to MD   If spitting up frequently and in significant volume; if there is weight loss, increasing constipation, or signs of illness requiring some evaluation

Emergency   Recurrent forceful vomiting, respiratory distress, or other serious, associated symptoms

Cross Reference   Breast-Feeding, Feeding of Infants, Vomiting

Inflammation of the pharynx caused by streptococcus

Etiology Group A beta-hemolytic streptococcus

Assessment The child usually has symptoms of fever, sore throat, and is generally "ill appearing". Lymph glands in the neck are often enlarged and tender. The child frequently has vomiting, headache, abdominal pain; tonsils are "beefy" red and often pus-covered. Tongue may look denuded ("strawberry tongue"). When rash is present, it feels like fine sandpaper.

Treatment/ Teaching Analgesics (ASA or acetaminophen) in appropriate dosage for age. Saline gargles. Fluids (cold drinks, ice chips, popsicles). Throat lozenges or topical anesthetic spray. Ice collar prn glandular swelling and discomfort. Antibiotic per MD. Child should be considered contagious until s/he has completed 24 hours of antibiotic therapy. A throat culture is indicated if a sore throat with fever and/or enlarged lymph glands has lasted 48 hours and is not subsiding.

Refer to MD For throat culture and treatment, for management of complications, (e.g., rheumatic fever or acute glomerulonephritis)

Emergency

Cross Reference Aspirin and Acetaminophen, Fever, Scarlet Fever or Scarlatina (Adult), Sore Throat, Swollen Glands (Adult)

Etiology

Assessment

Treatment/ Teaching

Refer to MD

Emergency

Cross Reference   Abdominal Pain (Adult), Abdominal Pain

Etiology

Assessment

Treatment/ Teaching

Refer to MD

Emergency

Cross Reference   Sunburn (Adult)

Abnormal enlargement of an area

Etiology   Trauma, infection, insect bites

Assessment   Determine if swelling generalized or localized. If the latter, determine if related to injury (e.g., fracture), to infectious process, or if allergic. For swelling around neck, jaw, and ear, determine exact localization. Mumps swelling occurs in front of and below the ear and above and below jawline; is a soft, tender swelling with low grade fever. With cervical lymphadenopathy, the swelling is below the jawline only, feels like firm hard knots and is usually associated with a URI or pharyngitis.

Treatment/
Teaching   **Injury:** Cold compresses or ice pack, elevation of extremity.

Cervical lymphadenopathy: Increase fluid intake. Aspirin or acetaminophen prn discomfort or fever. Ice collar prn discomfort. Watch for signs of infection in gland (increased swelling, tenderness, streaking).

Insect bites: see cross reference card.

Refer to MD   For fracture, suspected severe injury, allergic or infectious reaction to insect bites; any joint swelling, intermittent swelling in groin, or painless, gradual swelling in scrotum; for chronic, nonresolving lymphadenopathy

Emergency   Generalized swelling (can be allergic reaction or related to kidney, liver, or heart disease); swelling in groin or scrotum accompanied by pain, (e.g., testicular torsion or incarcerated hernia)

Cross
Reference   Allergic Reaction (Adult), Aspirin and Acetaminophen, Fractures or Dislocations (Adult), Ice Collar (Glossary), Inguinal or Scrotal Swelling, Mumps (Adult)

Process of and symptoms associated with eruption of primary teeth

Etiology

Assessment First tooth usually appears around 5 to 7 months of age, but this is variable. Drooling and chewing usually start at 3 months and are not reliable signs of teething. When teething begins, gums swell and become reddened and purplish over the area where the tooth will erupt. Lower incisors usually erupt 1st, followed by upper central, lateral incisors, 1st molars, canines, and 2nd molars. There may be 1° to 2° of temperature elevation during teething, but not a high fever. Teething is often accompanied by irritability. When some teeth erupt, there may be an associated release of serosanguinous fluid.

Treatment/ Teaching Aspirin or acetaminophen in dose appropriate to age; cold teething ring, popsicle; tea bag teether (see glossary); brandy or other alcohol rubbed directly on gums; local teething lotions

Refer to MD For excessive irritability with lethargy, high fever, or poor appetite

Emergency

Cross Reference Aspirin and Acetaminophen, Crying and Irritability, Tea Bag Teether (Glossary)

Guidelines for routine tetanus immunization schedule and for tetanus booster secondary to injury

Etiology

Assessment

Treatment/ Teaching

Routine Tetanus Immunization Schedule
DPT: 6 weeks, 4 months, 9 months, 2 years, and 5 years of age.
DT booster: Age 5 to 10 years with complete DPT series history.
TD booster*: Over 10 years of age with history of complete DPT series and no booster within the past 5 to 10 years.

Guidelines for Injury
With history of DPT series but no recent booster (i.e., within past 5 years), child should be seen within 72 hours of injury for injection.

See immediately if no previous tetanus immunization.

*TD booster (tetanus, diphtheria): only preparation available for diphtheria booster that is given on same schedule

Refer to MD   For injection

Emergency

Cross Reference   Bites, Animal and Human; Immunization Information, Lacerations

Etiology

Assessment

Treatment/ Teaching

Refer to MD

Emergency

Cross Reference   Tooth Avulsion (Adult)

Guidelines for caring for umbilical cord and umbilicus of newborn

Etiology

Assessment   Determine if there is a problem. Does the cord appear wet or dry? Is it oozing blood or foul-smelling discharge? Is the area red, swollen, purulent? Does the umbilicus bulge when the infant cries? Is fever present?

Treatment/ Teaching   Until the cord dries, may cleanse cord stump ONCE daily with alcohol. Cord drops off because of bacterial decomposition; the more sterile it is, the longer it will remain attached. May bathe baby, but don't soak for prolonged periods. Dry cord well after bath. Keep diapers and plastic pants pulled below the umbilicus until dry. Normally, the cord stump drops off between 7 to 21 days of age. A small amount of bloody oozing is common at that time. This can cause parents undue worry. Umbilical hernia (a protuberance of the umbilicus when the baby strains or cries) is a common condition that usually resolves by itself; there is no need to bind or tape the umbilicus.

Refer to MD   For active persistent bleeding from umbilicus, evaluation of umbilical hernia

Emergency   Signs of infection (presence of fever, inflamed swollen skin around umbilicus, purulent discharge)

Cross Reference   Abdominal Swelling

Guidelines for evaluating pediatric urinary problems

Etiology   Infection, irritation, pinworms, urinary retention

Assessment   Determine presence or absence of fever; frequency, urgency or painful urination; abdominal pain, flank pain; irritability; vomiting; hematuria (all are indicative of a UTI). In the younger child, unexplained intermittent fever is often the only sign. If dysuria is only symptom, ask about bubble bath or detergent use in bath water, hygiene, evidence of pinworms.

Treatment/ Teaching   If child unable to void, encourage child to urinate in warm sitz bath. Urge fluids. Do not take antibiotic before being seen by MD.

Refer to MD   If febrile, presence of frequency or urgency, abdominal pain

Emergency   High fever, flank pain, appears toxic, unable to urinate despite sitz bath

Cross Reference   Bed Wetting, Fever, Genitalia Problems, Pinworms

Guidelines for treatment of vaginal discharge in young girls and infants

Etiology   Normal, infection, trauma, foreign body, pinworms

Assessment   Determine if girl is menstruating or prepubertal, presence of foul odor, pain, itching, labial redness, swelling or sores, color of discharge and volume. Determine possibility of foreign body, trauma, history of intercourse or sexual abuse. See if irritation may be due to bubble bath, related to wearing diapers, or poor hygiene.

**Treatment/
Teaching**   Expect small amount of white vaginal discharge occasionally tinged with blood in the newborn. Sitz bath. Good hygiene. Expect small amount of mucoid, asymptomatic vaginal discharge in pubertal girls.

Refer to MD   For bloody discharge, foul odor, or pain; on routine basis for persistent discharge

Emergency   Evidence of sexual abuse, rape, or penetrating foreign body

**Cross
Reference**   Genitalia Problems

Etiology	Illness, ingestion of toxic substance, head or abdominal injury, side effect of medications, food poisoning, obstruction
Assessment	Rely on history and ancillary symptoms. Determine onset, duration, quantity, if projectile, type and color of vomitus, history of ingestion, exposure to illness (other family members spontaneously ill with same symptoms), history of injury to head or abdomen. Determine state of hydration (e.g., frequency of urine output, quantity of fluid intake), presence of other symptoms (e.g., diarrhea, fever, abdominal pain, headache, etc.). Does child appear toxic?
Treatment/ Teaching	Nothing PO for 2 hours after last emesis. Then sips of clear fluids every 20 to 30 minutes for 2 hours. Can use Pedialyte in infants, Gatorade, flat cola or 7-Up, ice chips, popsicles in older child. **Gradually** increase the amount given. After 2 hours, can give 1 oz every 20 to 30 minutes. After 24 hours without vomiting, resume breast-feeding or slowly resume other foods. If diarrhea, see cross reference card. Suppositories usually not used in infants, only with specific orders from MD. Have mother call back if vomiting persists or child develops signs of dehydration.
Refer to MD	If dehydration present (urination less than every 6 to 8 hours), high fever, severe headache or stiff neck, severe abdominal pain, persistent vomiting despite home treatment, poison ingestion, history of injury, blood in vomitus
Emergency	Severe pain, extreme lethargy, unresponsiveness
Cross Reference	Abdominal Pain, Dehydration, Diarrhea, Pyloric Stenosis

A whistling sound on expiration resulting from bronchial narrowing

Etiology   Asthma, aspiration of foreign body, bronchitis, allergies, heart disease, viral bronchiolitis (occurs from age 2 months to 3 years)

Assessment   Determine if child aspirated something (e.g., peanuts, popcorn, carrots, coins, safety pins, etc.), presence of upper respiratory infection, history of allergies or asthma; history of heart disease; if this is the first episode. Determine degree of distress (retracting, cyanotic, using neck and abdominal muscles to breathe), severity compared to previous episodes, if child taking medication for asthma and if it is offering any relief, quantity of fluid intake, presence of ancillary symptoms (e.g., fever).

Treatment/ Teaching   Increase clear fluid intake. Vaporizer (cool mist preferred). Child's usual asthma medications in the usual dosages. Call back if distress increases or if no improvement.

Refer to MD   If possibility of aspiration, if not improving with usual medications, if episode as severe as previous ones requiring injections and/or hospitalization, if no relief with home treatment

Emergency   Severe respiratory distress (i.e., fighting for air, retracting, cyanotic, using accessory muscles, unable to retain fluids)

Cross Reference   Common Cold, Cough

ANTIBIOTICS: Oral preparations for simple infections; dosage will vary significantly with serious infections.

Drug	How Supplied	Usual Dose
Amoxicillin	Suspension: 125 mg/5 cc	20–40 mg/kg/24 hours; given q8h or tid
Ampicillin	Tablet: 250 mg	80 mg/kg/24 hours; one q6h or qid
Cephradine	Suspension: 250 mg/5 cc Capsules: 250 or 500 mg	50–100 mg/kg/24 hours given q6h or qid
Dicloxacillin	Suspension: 62.5 mg/cc Capsules: 250 mg	25–75 mg/kg/24 hours given qid
Erythromycin	Tablet: 250 mg Chewable Tablet: 200 mg	30–50 mg/kg/24 hours given q6h or qid taken on an empty stomach
Erythromycin Ethylsuccinate	Suspension: 200 mg/5 cc 400 mg/5 cc	30–50 mg/kg/24 hours given q6h or qid given bid with food
LipoGantrisin	Suspension: 1,000 mg/5 cc	100–150 mg/kg/24 hours given bid
Potassium Phenoxymethyl Penicillin (Pen VK)	Suspension: 250 mg (400,000 U)/5cc Tablet: 250 mg	25,000–50,000 U/kg/24 hours 125–250 mg q6h or qid (200,000–400,000 U)
Nystatin	Suspension: 100,000 U/cc Tablet: 500,000 U	1 cc each side of mouth (2 cc total) qid, between feedings, on an empty stomach
Sulfamethoxazole	Liquid: 500 mg/5 cc Tablet: 500 mg	60 mg/kg/24 hours given qid

Trimethoprim-Sulfamethaxazole (Bactrim or Septra)
Tablet: 80 mg trimethoprim, 400 mg sulfamethoxazole
Liquid: ½ tablet = 5 cc

½ cc/kg q12h

KG(lb)	Tsp	Tab
10(22)	1(5 cc)	½
20(44)	2(10 cc)	1
30(66)	3(15 cc)	1½
40(88)	4(20 cc)	2

Tetracycline
(do not use in children
under 8 years of age)

ANTIEMETICS: to control nausea and vomiting

Drug	How Supplied	Usual Dose
Promethazine (Phenergan) Can cause sedation	Suppositories: 12.5 mg, 25 mg, 50 mg	0.25–0.5 mg/kg/q4-6h
Trimethobenzamide (Tigan) May cause sedation, neurologic effects, hypersensitivity	Suppositories: 100 mg, 200 mg Capsules: 100 mg, 250 mg	7–20 mg/kg/24 hours; divided into 4 doses

ANTIHISTAMINES, DECONGESTANTS, EXPECTORANTS, ANTITUSSIVES, ASTHMA MEDICATIONS: Antihistamines and decongestants are usually not indicated under 4 months of age. Recommend saline nasal aspirations or ⅛% Neo-Synephrine.

Drug	How Supplied	Usual Dose	
Tripolidine Hydrochloride & Pseudoephedrine Hydrochloride (Actifed) May cause drowsiness or stimulation Use: allergic or vasomotor rhinitis	Tablet or Syrup: one strength	**Age** 4 months-2 years 2-4 years 4-6 years 6-12 years	**Dose** ¼ tsp tid-qid ½ tsp tid-qid ¾ tsp tid-qid 1 tsp tid-qid
Diphenhydramine (Benadryl) Antihistamine; may cause drowsiness, excitation, dry mucous membranes Use: allergic rhinitis, allergic reaction to insect bites, itching	Elixir: 12.5 mg/5 cc	5 mg/kg/24 hours up to a maximum of 300 mg given tid or qid Infant: ½ tsp (6.75 mg) tid-qid Child: 1 tsp (12.5 mg) tid-qid	
Diphenhydramine & 5% Alcohol (Benylin) Antihistamine; may cause drowsiness, excitation, dry mucous membranes Use: mild allergic reaction, irritative cough	Syrup: one strength	**Age** 2-6 years 6-12 years over 12 years	**Dose** ½-1 tsp qid 1 tsp qid 2 tsp qid

ANTIHISTAMINES, DECONGESTANTS, EXPECTORANTS, ANTITUSSIVES, ASTHMA MEDICATIONS: Antihistamines and decongestants are usually not indicated under 4 months of age. Recommend saline nasal aspirations or $\frac{1}{8}$% Neo-Synephrine.

Drug	How Supplied	Usual Dose	
Chlorpheniramine Maleate (Chlor-Trimeton, Corciden, Triaminic) Antihistamine; may cause drowsiness, excitation, dry mucous membranes Use: allergic rhinitis, allergic conjunctivitis, urticaria	Tablet: 4 mg Extentab: 8 mg & 12 mg Elixir: 2 mg/5 cc	**Age** Infant-2 years 2-12 years over 12 years	**Dose** ¼ tsp tid-qid ½-1 tsp or ½ tab (2 mg) tid or qid 1 tab (4 mg) qid or 1 extentab (8 mg) bid .35 mg/kg/24 hours given tid-qid
Guaifenesin, Codeine, and Alcohol (Cheracol) Prescription; may cause CNS depression Use: cough suppressant, pain	Syrup: Guaifenesin 100 mg/5 cc Codeine 10 mg/5 cc Alcohol 3% Available OTC without Codeine (see 2/G)	**Age** 2-6 years 6-12 years	**Dose** ½ tsp qid or only ½ tsp hs ½-1 tsp qid
Dextromethorphan (Robitussin DM, Benylin DM, Cheracol D, etc.) May cause nausea and dizziness Use: nonnarcotic cough suppressant	Syrup: 10 mg/5 cc in 5% Alcohol	1 mg/kg/24 hours; give in 3-4 divided doses	
Brompheniramine Maleate, Phenylephrine Hydrochloride, Alcohol 2.3% (Dimetapp) Antihistamine, decongestant; may cause drowsiness or stimulation Use: allergic or vasomotor rhinitis	Elixir Extentab	**Age** 1-6 months 7 months-2 years 2-4 years 4-12 years over 12 years	**Dose** ¼ tsp tid-qid ½ tsp tid-qid ¾ tsp tid-qid 1 tsp tid-qid 1-2 tsp tid-qid or 1 extentab bid

ANTIHISTAMINES, DECONGESTANTS, EXPECTORANTS, ANTITUSSIVES, ASTHMA MEDICATIONS: Antihistamines and decongestants are usually not indicated under 4 months of age. Recommend saline nasal aspirations or $\frac{1}{8}$% Neo-Synephrine.

Drug	How Supplied	Usual Dose	
Cyproheptadine Hydrochloride (Periactin) Antihistamine; do not give to children less than 2 years of age. May cause drowsiness excitability, dry mucous membranes Use: allergic rhinitis, allergic conjunctivitis, urticaria, allergic reaction to insect bites, itching	Liquid: 2 mg/5 cc Tablet: 4 mg	0.25 mg/kg/24 hours **Age** 2-6 years 7-14 years	**Dose** 1 tsp or ½ tab (2 mg) tid 2 tsp or 1 tab (4 mg) tid
Guaifenesin (Robitussin, 2/G) Expectorant; lubricates inflamed membranes Do not use prior to surgery (may decrease platelet adhesiveness)	Syrup: Guiafenesin 100 mg/5 ml Alcohol 3.5%	12 mg/kg/24 hours given qid **Weight (age)** 15-25 lb (6 months-2 years) 25-30 lb (2-3 years) 30-60 lb (3-5 years) over 5 years	**Dose** ¼ tsp qid ½ tsp qid ¾ tsp qid 1 tsp qid
Pseudoephedrine (Sudafed) Decongestant; may cause stimulation Use: rhinitis	Elixir: 30 mg/5 cc Tablet: 30-60 mg	**Age** 4 months-2 years 2-4 years 4-6 years 6-12 years	**Dose** ¼ tsp tid-qid ½ tsp tid-qid ¾ tsp tid-qid 1 tsp tid-qid

ASTHMA PREPARATIONS (to control wheezing and bronchospasm)

FOR ANY QUESTIONS REGARDING USE OF THESE DRUGS, CONTACT PHYSICIAN

Drug	How Supplied	Usual Dose
Metaproterenol (Alupent) Not approved for use under 2 years of age Use: Brochodilator for bronchial asthma and for reversible bronchospasm associated with bronchitis	Syrup: 10 mg/5 cc	0.25-0.5 mg/kg/dose q5-6h Do not exceed 1 tsp per dose

ASTHMA PREPARATIONS (to control wheezing and bronchospasm)

Drug	How Supplied	Usual Dose
Theophylline Preparations May cause nausea, vomiting, tachycardia, CNS stimulation Use: asthma		
(Slophyllin)	Syrup: 80 mg/15 cc Tablets: 100 mg, 200 mg Gyrocaps: 60 mg, 125 mg, 250 mg	5 mg/kg/q6h
(Slophyllin GG)	Syrup: (per 15 cc) Theophylline 150 mg Guaifenesin 90 mg Capsule: same dosage	
(Marax)	Tablets: Theophylline 130 mg Ephedrine 25 mg Atarax 10 mg Liquid: (per 5 cc) Theophylline 32.5 mg Ephedrine 25 mg Atarax 2.5 mg	
(Aminophylline)	Tablets: 100 mg, 200 mg	
(Theolair)	Tablets: 125 mg, 250 mg	
(Theodur)	Tablets: 100 mg, 200 mg 300 mg	

ANTIPARASITICS: For treatment of parasites e.g., lice, scabies, pinworms

Drug	How Supplied	Usual Dose
A-200 Pyrinate Not used in individuals allergic to ragweed Use: control of lice	Liquid Gel	1 application for 10 minutes may repeat but no more than 2 doses/24 hours
Crotamiton (Eurax) Can cause skin irritation Use: only used in cases of Kwell-resistant scabies	Cream Lotion	Apply from the chin down; bathe before and after using (apply at hs for 3 days) (If child is less than 2 years of age, use Sulfur 10% in Heb cream water base)
Gamma Benzene Hexachloride (Kwell) Use: scabies, lice Do not use if skin lesions are present or if client is under 5 years of age	Lotion Shampoo	Bathe and apply to affected skin, wash off completely in 8-12 hours Use as a shampoo then rinse out Repeat only under the direction of the MD

ANTIPARASITICS: For treatment of parasites e.g., lice, scabies, pinworms

Drug	How Supplied	Usual Dose
RID Not used in individuals allergic to ragweed Use: control of lice	Liquid	1 application for 10 minutes; may repeat PRN but no more than 2 doses/24 hours
Meleandazole (Vermox) Don't use in pregnant women or children under 2 years Use: pinworms	Tablets	1 chewable tablet, 1 time; may repeat once in 10 days; check with MD for treatment of other parasites

ANTIPYRETICS/ANALGESICS: refer to Aspirin and Acetaminophen card in Pediatric Section

GASTROINTESTINAL MEDS: Meds commonly used to reduce GI spasm and vomiting; to replace electrolytes and normal intestinal bacteria

Drug	How Supplied	Usual Dose
Lactobacillus (Bacid) Use: diarrhea related to antibiotic therapy	Capsules	0-2 years: ½ capsule in food qid 2+ years: 1 capsule with food qid
Dicyclomine Hydrochloride (Bentyl) Use: colic (antispasmodic)	Elixir (always order half-strength): 10 mg/tsp	Infant: 2.5-4 cc 10 minutes before meals during fussy periods (do not exceed 4 doses/day) 0.5-1 mg/kg/day q6-8h
Oral electrolyte solution with dextrose (Pedialyte) Use: diarrhea and vomiting Generally not enjoyed by children over 18-20 months (try Gatorade)	Liquid: 32 oz cans 8 oz bottles	Give ad lib for 24-36 hours while child is symptomatic
Promethazine Hydrochloride (Phenergan) Use: intractible vomiting	Suppositories: 12.5 mg, 25 mg, 50 mg	Children: 0.25 mg/kg/q6-8h never exceed adult dose (12.5-25 mg/q3-6h) If suppository needs to be halved, cut lengthwise only. After insertion, turn crossways in the rectum to help prevent expulsion
Trimethobenzamide (Tigan) Use: intractible vomiting	Suppositories: 100 mg, 200 mg with benzocaine	7-20 mg/kg/24 hours given qid

VITAMINS AND MINERALS: Used as dietary supplements

Drug	How Supplied	Usual Dose
Ferrous Gluconate (Fer in Sol) Iron preparations are better absorbed if taken 10 minutes ac with high-Vit C juice (orange or Tang)	Elixir: 7 mg/cc Drops: 15 mg/.6 cc, 25 mg/cc	Maintenance: 2-3 mg/kg/day Therapeutic: 6-9 mg/kg/day given tid
Fluoride	Drops: 0.25 mg/drop Tablet: 1 mg	0-2 years: 0.25 mg/day 2-3 years: 0.5 mg/day 3+ years: 1 mg/day
Poly Vi Sol (Vit A,B,C,D,E)	Liquid Tablet	1 cc or 1 tablet/day
Tri Vi Flor or **Poly Vi Flor**	Chewable Tablet: Fluoride 0.5 mg, 1 mg Liquid: Fluoride 0.25 mg, 0.5 mg/cc	1 cc or 1 tablet/day
Tri Vi Sol (Vit A,C,D)	Tablet Liquid	1 cc or 1 tablet/day
Tri Vi Sol or **Poly Vi Sol with Iron**	Tablet: Iron 12 mg Liquid: Iron 10 mg/cc	1 cc or 1 tablet/day

APPENDIX 1:
COMMONLY PRESCRIBED OVER-THE-COUNTER DRUGS

ACNE PREPARATIONS

Name and Manufacturer	Active Ingredients	Major Indications	Special Instructions
Acnaveen (Cooper Care) bar	Sulfur 2% Salicylic acid 2% Colloidal oatmeal	Causes mild peeling & drying, reduces blackheads, whiteheads	Discontinue if skin irritation
Fostex (Westwood) bar	Sulfur 2% Salicylic acid 2%	Causes mild peeling and drying; reduces blackheads, whiteheads	Discontinue if skin irritation
*__Benoxyl__ (Stiefel) lotion	Benzoyl peroxide 5%, 10%	Causes mild peeling & drying	1–3% are hypersensitive
*__Clearasil B.P.__ (Vicks) lotion, cream	Benzoyl peroxide 5%, 10%	Reduces P. acnes (Bactericidal)	Start with 5% preparation and use 1–2 times daily unless excessive stinging
*__Oxy-5, Oxy-10__ (Norcliff-Thayer) lotion	Benzoyl peroxide 5%, 10%	Reduces P. acnes (Bactericidal)	

*Drug of choice

ANTACIDS: Liquid better than tablets unless tablets chewed well and swallowed with water.

Name and Manufacturer	Active Ingredients	Major Indications	Special Instructions
Alternagel (Stuart) liquid	Aluminum hydroxide	Acid indigestion, heartburn	Neither constipating nor causes diarrhea
Gelusil (Parke-Davis) tablet, liquid	Aluminum hydroxide Magnesium hydroxide	Acid indigestion, heartburn	Magnesium may cause diarrhea

ANTACIDS: Liquid better than tablets unless tablets chewed well and swallowed with water.

Name and Manufacturer	Active Ingredients	Major Indications	Special Instructions
Maalox (Rorer) tablet, liquid	Aluminum hydroxide Magnesium hydroxide	Acid indigestion, heartburn	Magnesium may cause diarrhea
Digel (Plough) tablet, liquid	Magnesium carbonate Magnesium hydroxide Simethicone	Acid indigestion, heartburn, antiflatulent	May cause diarrhea
Maalox Plus (Rorer)	Aluminum hydroxide Magnesium hydroxide Simethicone	Acid indigestion, heartburn, antiflatulent	May cause diarrhea
Mylanta, Mylanta II (Stuart) tablet, liquid	Aluminum hydroxide Magnesium hydroxide Simethicone	Acid indigestion, heartburn, antiflatulent	May cause diarrhea
Rolaids (Warner Lambert) tablet	Dihydroxyaluminum Sodium Carbonate	Acid indigestion, heartburn	May cause diarrhea
Tums (Norcliff-Thayer) tablet	Calcium Carbonate	Acid indigestion, heartburn	Calcium may cause constipation—good in pregnancy due to calcium content

SIGNIFICANT DRUG INTERACTIONS: Give antacids at least 2 hours before or 1 hour after the following medications to prevent reduced absorption: tetracycline, digoxin, digitoxin, chlorpromazine (Thorazine), indomethacin (Indocin). Antacids can increase levodopa (Laradopa) absorption up to 3 times and make client toxic.

ANTIFUNGAL

Name and Manufacturer	Active Ingredients	Major Indications	Special Instructions
Cruex (Pharmacraft) cream, powder, spray powder	Undecylenic acid 2.5-10%	"Jock" itch, tinea cruris	Discontinue if skin irritation develops
Desenex (Pharmacraft) foam, liquid, ointment, powder	Undecylenic acid 2.5-10%	Tinea pedis (athlete's foot), tinea capitis, tinea corporis (ringworm)	Discontinue if skin irritation develops
*Tinactin (Schering) cream, powder, powder aerosol, liquid aerosol, solution	Tolnaftate 1%	Tinea pedis, tinea capitis, tinea corporis, tinea cruris	Very nonsensitizing

ANTIFUNGAL

Name and Manufacturer	Active Ingredients	Major Indications	Special Instructions
Whitfield's Ointment (various)	Benxoic acid 6% Salicylic acid 3%	Tinea pedis, tinea capitis, tinea corporis, tinea cruris	Discontinue if skin irritation develops

*Drug of choice

ANTIPYRETICS—ASPIRIN PREPARATIONS: Antipyretic, analgesic, antiinflammatory

Name and Manufacturer	Active Ingredients	Major Indications	Special Instructions
Anacin (Whitehall) tablets	Aspirin 400 mg Caffeine		10 mg/kg/dose Normally do not use in viral illness
Anacin Maximum Strength (Whitehall) tablets	Aspirin 500 mg Caffeine		
Bayer Aspirin (Glenbrook) tablets, children's tablets time-release	Aspirin 325 mg Aspirin 81 mg Aspirin 650 mg		
Excedrin (Bristol Myers) capsules	Aspirin 250 mg Acetaminophen 250 mg Caffeine		
Excedrin PM (Bristol Myers) capsules	Aspirin 250 mg Acetaminophen 250 mg Pyrilamine maleate		Antihistamine causing drowsiness, dry mouth
St. Joseph's Aspirin (Plough) tablets	Aspirin 325 mg		
St. Joseph's Aspirin for Children (Plough) chewable tablet	Aspirin 81 mg		10 mg/kg/dose Normally do not use in viral illness

DRUG INTERACTIONS: Avoid aspirin with probenecid, sulfinpyrazone, warfarin, sulfonylureas (oral antidiabetic medications).

ANTIPYRETICS—ACETAMINOPHEN PREPARATIONS: Antipyretic, analgesic

Name and Manufacturer	Active Ingredients	Major Indications	Special Instructions
Anacin III (Whitehall) tablets	Acetaminophen 500 mg Caffeine		10 mg/kg/dose
Datril (Bristol Myers)	Acetaminophen 325 mg		
Datril 500 (Norcliff-Thayer) liquid	Acetaminophen 120 mg/2.5 ml		
Tylenol (McNeil) chewable tablets, elixir, drops, tablets, extra-strength capsules	Acetaminophen 80 mg 160 mg/5 ml 100 mg/ml 325 mg 500 mg		

ACETAMINOPHEN CAUTION: Chronic use of 5 gm/day (10 extra strength capsules) can cause liver toxicity, especially if an alcohol user.

ANTISEPTICS

Name and Manufacturer	Active Ingredients	Major Indications	Special Instructions
Polysporin (Burroughs Wellcome) ointment	Bacitracin Polysporin	Topical antibiotic	Avoid neomycin— can cause hypersensitivity
Campho-Phenique (Winthrop) liquid	Phenol	Antiseptic, local anesthetic for cold sores/ cankersores	ADA does not recommend— can cause tissue damage
Blistex (Blistex) ointment	Camphor Phenol spirits of ammonia	Topical counterirritant	ADA does not recommend, no proven efficacy

COLD/ALLERGY/ANTIHISTAMINE PREPARATIONS

Name and Manufacturer	Active Ingredients	Major Indications	Special Instructions
Antihistamine			
Benylin (Parke-Davis) liquid	Diphenhydramine 12.5 mg/5 ml	Allergy, pruritus, cough	1.25 mg/kg/dose for children for allergy. Remind patients of additional drowsiness with sedatives or alcohol
Chlor-Trimeton (Schering) tablet, liquid	Chlorpheniramine 2 mg/5 ml	Allergy, colds	.35 mg/kg/day in 4 doses
Decongestant Only			
Afrin (Schering) nose drops, spray, pediatric drops	Oxymetazoline	Congested nose, sinusitis	
Neo-Synephrine (Winthrop) nose drops, spray	Phenylephrine	Congested nose, sinusitis	
Sudafed (Burroughs-Wellcome) tablets, syrup	Pseudoephedrine 30 mg Pseudoephedrine 30 mg/5 ml		Use 2 tabs qid if necessary Peds: 5-8 mg/kg/day in 4-6 doses
Antihistamine/Decongestant Combinations Colds/Allergy			
Chlor-Trimeton Decongestant (Schering) tablet	*Chlorpheniramine 4 mg **Pseudoephedrine 60 mg	Congested nose, sinusitis, allergy	As directed
Coricidin D (Schering) tablet	*Chlorpheniramine 2 mg **Phenylpropanolamine Aspirin	Congested nose, sinusitis, allergy	As directed
Contac (Menley & James) time capsule	*Chlorpheniramine **Phenylpropanolamine	Congested nose, sinusitis, allergy	As directed

COLD/ALLERGY/ANTIHISTAMINE PREPARATIONS

Name and Manufacturer	Active Ingredients	Major Indications	Special Instructions
Antitussives			
2/G (Dow) liquid	Guaifenesin 100 mg/5 ml	Expectorant	Peds: 12 mg/kg/ day in 6 doses
Robitussin (Robins) liquid	Guaifenesin 100 mg/5 ml	Expectorant	Peds: 12 mg/kg/ day in 6 doses
Cheracol-D (Upjohn) liquid	Dextromethorphan 10 mg/5 ml Guaifenesin	Cough suppressant, expectorant	Peds: 1 mg/kg/day in 3-4 doses
Robitussin DM (Robins)	Dextromethorphan 10 mg/5 ml Guaifenesin	Cough suppressant, expectorant	Peds: 1 mg/kg/day in 3-4 doses
Novahistine Cough Formula (Dow) liquid	Dextromethorphan 10 mg/5 ml Guaifenesin	Cough suppressant, expectorant	Peds: 1 mg/kg/day in 3-4 doses
Sorbituss (Dalin) liquid	Dextromethrophan 10 mg/5 ml Guaifenesin	Cough suppressant, expectorant Sugar-free, alcohol-free	
Triaminic Expectorant (Dorsey) liquid	Guaifenesin 100 mg/5 ml *Phenylpropanolamine, **Pheniramine, Pyrilamine	Expectorant, decongestant, antihistamine, (cough/cold)	

*Avoid antihistamines in narrow-angle glaucoma (using anticholinesterase), most asthmatics, urinary retention. Remind clients of additional drowsiness with sedatives or alcohol.
Oral decongestants (phenylpropanolamine, phenylephrine, pseudoephedrine) should not be used in clients with diabetes mellitus, hypertension, hyperthyroidism, or ischemic heart disease except on advice of physician. **Do not use with MAO inhibitors, guanethidine (Ismelin)

DANDRUFF CONTROL

Name and Manufacturer	Active Ingredients	Major Indications	Special Instructions
Sebulex Conditioning Formula and Medicated Shampoo (Westwood)	Salicylic acid 2% Sulfur 2%	Antiseborrheic	

DANDRUFF CONTROL

Name and Manufacturer	Active Ingredients	Major Indications	Special Instructions
Sebutone (Westwood) shampoo	Salicylic acid 2% Sulfur 2% Tar 0.5%	Antiseborrheic	Tar may discolor blond or bleached hair
Selsun Blue (Abbott) shampoo	Selenium sulfide 1%	Antiseborrheic	May cause skin irritation—don't use on broken skin
Tegrin (Block) cream, lotion, shampoo	Allantoin 0.2% (cream, lotion) Coal tar 5%	Psoriasis	Tar may discolor blond or bleached hair

ELECTROLYTE SOLUTIONS—ORAL (Infants and Children)

Name and Manufacturer	Active Ingredients	Major Indications	Special Instructions
Lytren (Mead Johnson) liquid	Electrolytes 9 calories/oz	Diarrhea, vomiting	Preferred by many pediatricians— better formulation
Pedialyte (Ross) liquid	Electrolytes 6 calories/oz	Diarrhea, vomiting	
Gatorade liquid, powder	Electrolytes Carbohydrates	Older children	Available in supermarkets

EYEDROPS

Name and Manufacturer	Active Ingredients	Major Indications	Special Instructions
Murine (Abbott) drops	Benzalkonium chloride Glycerin	Artificial tears	
Visine (Leeming) drops	Tetrahydrozoline hydrochloride Preservatives Buffer	Decongestant	Do not use in narrow-angle glaucoma Short-term use only

HEMORRHOID PREPARATIONS

Name and Manufacturer	Active Ingredients	Major Indications	Special Instructions
Lanacaine (Combe) cream	Benzocaine 6% Chlorothymol Resorcinol	Local anesthetic	Resorcinol not recommended
Nupercainal (Ciba) ointment, suppositories	Dibucaine 1%	Local anesthetic	Discontinue if hypersensitivity develops
Tronolane (Abbott) cream, suppositories	Pramoxine 1%	Local anesthetic	Discontinue if hypersensitivity develops
Tucks (Parke-Davis) pads, cream, ointment	Hamamelis Water 50%	Astringent, external protectant	Hemorrhoids

LAXATIVES

Name and Manufacturer	Active Ingredients	Major Indications	Special Instructions
Colace (Mead Johnson) capsules, liquid	Docusate 100 mg/capsule	Stool softener	Do not take with mineral oil
Glycerin (various) suppositories	Glycerin (pediatric and adult sizes)	Stimulant (local)	
Metamucil (Searle) powder, packets	Psyllium mucilloid	Bulk-forming, laxative	
Milk of Magnesia (Philips Roxane) liquid	Magnesium hydroxide	Saline laxative	Contraindicated in renal dysfunction or reduced CNS function

LICE PREPARATIONS

Name and Manufacturer	Active Ingredients	Major Indications	Special Instructions
A-200 Pyrinate (Norcliff-Thayer) liquid, gel	Pyrethrins 0.33% Piperonyl butoxide 4% Kerosene 5%	Lice, scabies	Kerosene is toxic on ingestion or inhalation
RID (Pfipharmics) shampoo	Pyrethrins 0.3% Piperonyl butoxide 3% Petroleum distillate 1.29%	Lice (head only)	Petroleum distillate is toxic on ingestion or inhalation

ORAL MUCOSAL ANALGESICS

Name and Manufacturer	Active Ingredients	Major Indications	Special Instructions
Anbesol (Whitehall) liquid, gel	Benzocaine 6.3%	Local anesthetic	Discontinue if hypersensitivity
Gly-Oxide (Marion) liquid	Carbamide peroxide	Cleansing effect, decreased inflammation due to oxygen release	
Orabase (Hoyt) paste	Protective base (pectin, gelatin, etc.)	Protectant	
Orabase with Benzocaine (Hoyt) paste	Benzocaine in protective base	Protectant, local anesthetic	Discontinue if hypersensitivity

TOPICAL ANTIINFLAMMATORY/ANTIPRURITIC/ASTRINGENT PREPARATIONS

Name and Manufacturer	Active Ingredients	Major Indications	Special Instructions
Calamine Lotion (various)		Astringent	
Caladryl Lotion (Parke-Davis)	Diphenhydramine Calamine	Antipruritic, antihistamine, astringent	Discontinue if hypersensitivity to diphenhydramine
CaldeCORT (Pharmacraft) cream, spray	Hydrocortisone 0.5%	Antiinflammatory	
Cortaid (Upjohn) cream	Hydrocortisone 0.5%	Antiinflammatory	
ClearAid (Squibb) cream, lotion, ointment	Hydrocortisone 0.5%	Antiinflammatory	
Dermolate (Schering) cream, spray	Hydrocortisone 0.5%	Antiinflammatory	

Pharmaceutical References

American Pharmaceutical Association. *Handbook of Nonprescription Drugs*, 7th Edition. Washington, DC: 1982.
Boyd, J., ed. *Facts and Comparisons*, St. Louis: Lippincott, 1983.
Shirkey, H. *Pediatric Dosage Handbook*. Washington, DC: American Pharmaceutical Association. 1980.

C. Swenson, Pharm. D. *Pharmacy Affairs, Group Health Cooperative*

A very important aspect of telephone health care is the documentation of the telephone encounter. Documentation is important for a number of reasons

- To provide further care. The nurse may need to reestablish contact with the client.
- For continuity of care. The client can receive follow-up care for the problem.
- For legal protection. Clear and concise documentation validates the nurse's practice.

Sample documentation form for telephone consultation

TELEPHONE CONSULTATION FORM

GROUP HEALTH COOPERATIVE OF PUGET SOUND				
	TIME	PHONE(H)	(W)	
DATE	TIME	CALL RETURNED	(PT. ADDRESS)	
NAME		PHYSICIAN	MEDICAL CENTER	
M.H.#	MO./YR. OF BIRTH	SPECIALIST		
PRESENTING PROBLEM	TEMP:	ASSESSMENT & ADVICE		
	INITIALS			
ALLERGIES:	PREGNANT	Rx		
CHRONIC DISEASE:	☐ YES ☐ NO			
CURRENT MEDS:		SIGNATURE		
		CHECKED WITH		
PM-1301 (14-03510) 8/79	APPOINTMENT MADE: ☐ MD ☐ RN ☐ MX	SIGNATURE	INSERT IN CHART	INITIALS

ac	before meals
ad lib	as much as desired
A&D	vitamin A&D
AF	atrial fibrillation
ASA	aspirin
bid	twice daily
BM	bowel movement
C°	centigrade or Celsius
cc	cubic centimeter
CHF	congestive heart failure
CNS	central nervous system
COPD	chronic obstructive pulmonary disease
CPR	cardiopulmonary resuscitation
CTM	Chlor-Trimeton
CVA	cerebral vascular accident
DPT	Diphtheria/Pertussis/Tetanus
DT	delirium tremens
ETH	elixir of terpin hydrate
F°	Fahrenheit
FDA	Federal Drug Administration
2/G	name of cough suppressant
GI	gastrointestinal
gm	gram
gr	grain
GU	genitourinary
hs	hour of sleep (bedtime)
HCG	human chorionic gonadotropin
IUD	intrauterine device
I&D	incision & drainage
kg	kilogram
lb	pound
LMP	last menstrual period
mg	milligram
MI	myocardial infarction
mm	millimeter

MMR	Measles/Mumps/Rubella
Na	sodium
NTG	nitroglycerin
OPV	oral polio vaccine
OTC	over the counter
O_2	oxygen
oz	ounce
PAT	paroxysmal atrial tachycardia
PE	polyethylene
peds	pediatrics
per	through
PID	pelvic inflammatory disease
PO	by mouth
prn	as needed
PVC	premature ventricular contraction
PPD	purified protein derivative (test for tuberculosis)
qid	4 times daily
r/o	rule out
RUQ	right upper quadrant
SOB	shortness of breath
STAT	immediately
tid	3 times daily
Tb	tuberculosis
TSS	toxic shock syndrome
TUR	transurethral resection
tab	tablet
T&A	tonsilectomy & adenoidectomy
tbsp	tablespoon
tsp	teaspoon
U	unit
UA	urinalysis
URI	upper respiratory infection
UTI	urinary tract infection
VNA	Visiting Nurses Association
WBC	white blood count

Baking Soda Bath

Add a generous amount of baking soda (½ cup or more) to ½ tub of warm water.

Baking Soda Paste

A smooth paste made from baking soda and water. Useful for relieving itching secondary to chickenpox and insect bites.

Benadryl-Maalox Mix

A solution of equal parts of Benadryl Elixir and Maalox to be used as a mouthwash or gargle for the relief of pain of oral herpes infections.

Clear Liquids

Fluids that are transparent. These include water, carbonated beverages, clear fruit juices, broth, Gatorade, tea, Jello.

Cool Compresses

Cloths or towel soaked in cool water or ice water and wrung out. Change frequently as coolness disappears.

Cornstarch Bath

One handful of cornstarch added to a tub of tepid water or add ½ to 1 lb cornstarch to a pot of hot water then add to bath; soak about 15 minutes. Useful to relieve itching and irritation.

Cornstarch Paste

A smooth paste made from cornstarch and water. Apply to painful, burning rashes for a soothing effect. Particularly useful on a fiery diaper rash.

Diarrhea Diet (Adult)

Clear fluids for 12 to 24 hours (water, 7-Up or ginger ale, Gatorade, tea, or broth). If diarrhea has stopped, advance to selected solids, i.e., nonsweetened cereals of rice or corn, bread (not whole grain), macaroni, potatoes, rice, yellow vegetables (squash or carrots), light-colored fruits (apples or bananas), and meats. No dairy products for 3 to 6 days.

Diarrhea Diet (Pediatric)

Clear fluids for 12 to 24 hours (Gatorade, 7-Up or ginger ale, water, weak tea); Pedialyte for infants. When diarrhea has stopped, advance to soy formula diluted with **twice** the amount of water called for on the can; increase concentration to full strength over a 24-hour period, then advance to select solids as listed in the adult diet. Withhold dairy products for 3 to 6 days. If the child is not on formula, advance to rice cereal, bananas, yellow vegetables, clear fluids as listed for beverage after 24 hours on clear liquids.

Elevate

Raise above the level of the heart.

Honey-Lemon Cough Mix

Two parts honey to 1 part lemon juice. One part alcohol (brandy, rum, vodka, etc.) may be added if desired. The honey is soothing to the throat and also acts as an expectorant; the lemon juice helps reduce the viscosity of phlegm; and the alcohol is an antitussive. This may be taken by the teaspoonful as needed for cough by adults or older children. Infants and young children should use a ¼ tsp dose. Substitute corn syrup (light) for honey for children under 1 year of age (because of the possibility of botulism spores in honey, which can produce the disease in infants but do not affect older children and adults.).

Hot Packs

Cloths or towels soaked in hot water and wrung out. A plastic covering and then a hot water bottle may be put on top of the towel to prolong the heat. Usually used for 20-minute intervals.

Ice Collar

Place crushed ice in a plastic bag, cover with a towel and drape across the client's neck. Useful in reducing the discomfort of a sore throat or swollen glands. A wet dishtowel frozen around a large cylinder (e.g., can) also makes an effective collar.

Ice Massage

Wrap a cloth around a frozen juice can or put frozen juice can in a sock and roll the can over the muscle in spasm. The combination of cold and massage is often useful in reducing muscle spasm.

Ice Pack

Place crushed ice in a plastic bag and cover with a towel. Do not put ice directly on the skin (due to possibility of causing ice burn). Ice packs are usually used for 20-minute intervals.

Karo Water

One tbsp of **dark** Karo syrup to 3 oz of warm water. Useful as a laxative for infants.

Meat Tenderizer Paste

Half tsp of meat tenderizer to 2 tsp of water. Helpful to draw poison out of bee sting. For oral use if piece of meat aspirated, dissolve 1 tsp tenderizer in 8 oz warm water. Sip and gargle until meat can be dislodged.

Neo-Synephrine Pledget

A small piece of cotton soaked with Neo-Synephrine or other vasoconstricting nose drops. Insert the pledget into the nostril to help stop a nosebleed.

Night Air

Damp, cool, night air. Very useful in reversing croup and in decreasing wheezing.

Oatmeal Bath

Fill a thin cloth or the toe of an old nylon stocking with uncooked oatmeal flakes (about 1 cup), tie closed, and allow to float in a bathtub of tepid water. Or, cook the bag of oatmeal for ½ hour then squeeze the bag in warm bath water to extract the gelatinous starch. A bath in this solution is often useful to reduce vaginal itching.

Piggyback

To alternate therapeutic doses of ASA and acetaminophen every 2 hours to reduce fever that is not responding to the use of only 1 antipyretic.

Saline

Quarter tsp salt to 1 cup water.

Saline Gargle or Mouthwash

Quarter tsp salt to 1 cup water (warm or cool, whichever feels best).

Saline Nose Drops

Quarter tsp salt to 1 cup warm water. Use per dropper prn nasal congestion.

Sitz Bath

A shallow, warm tub bath usually lasting 20 minutes at a time. Useful for healing hemorrhoids, anal lesions, boils, and episiotomies.

Steamy Bathroom

A bathroom filled with steam from running hot water in tub or shower until the room is foggy. Often used for respiratory congestion, wheezing, and croup if a vaporizer is not accessible. The bathroom window can be opened partially to help simulate cold steam.

Tea Bag Teether

Brew a cup of tea. After steeping, wring out the tea bag and let it cool. Let the infant chew on the moist bag. The tannic acid in the tea helps reduce inflammation in gums.

Tepid Bath

Lukewarm water deep enough to cover client's legs. Splash water on trunk. Do not submerge child in water. Try to keep client in tub 20 to 30 minutes.

Urge Fluids

Refers to increasing clear fluid intake. For adults, this usually means an 8 oz glass/hour while awake, up to 6 to 8 glasses. Less for elderly clients or those with heart disease.

Vinegar Douche

1 tbsp of white vinegar to 1 quart tepid water. Helpful for yeast infections and other causes of vaginal itching.

American Academy of Pediatrics. *Report of the Committee on Infectious Disease*. Evanston, IL: American Academy of Pediatrics, 1982.

Dorland, W. *Dorland's Illustrated Medical Dictionary*. Philadelphia: Saunders, 1981.

Hoole, A., Greenberg, R., and Packard, C. *Client Care Guidelines for Nurse Practitioners*. Boston: Little, Brown, 1982.

Hudak, C., Redstone, P., Hakanson, N., and Suzuki, I. *Clinical Protocols*. Philadelphia: Lippincott, 1976.

Kempe, C., Silver, H., and Donough, O. *Current Pediatric Diagnosis and Treatment*. Los Altos, CA: Lange Medical Publications, 1982.

Krupp, M. and Chatton, M. *Current Medical Diagnosis and Treatment*. Los Altos, CA: Lange Medical Publications, 1982.

Leitch, C. and Tinker, R. *Primary Care*. Philadelphia: Davis, 1978.

Roper, N. *New American Pocket Dictionary*. New York: Churchill Livingston, 1978.

Stedman, T. *Stedman's Medical Dictionary*. Baltimore: Williams & Wilkins, 1982.